Controversies in Liver Transplantation - Recent Challenges and Future Perspectives

Edited by Dipesh Kumar Yadav

Published in London, United Kingdom

Controversies in Liver Transplantation - Recent Challenges and Future Perspectives
http://dx.doi.org/10.5772/intechopen.98029
Edited by Dipesh Kumar Yadav

Contributors
Federica Invernizzi, Marta Cilla, Santiago Rodríguez Villafuerte, Adilson Renato Veríssimo, Luis Geovanny Mochas, Fabian André Zurita, Julio Patricio Salazar, Dipesh Kumar Yadav, Rajesh Kumar Yadav, Tingbo Liang, Ana Fajreldines, Victoria Fornari, Marcelo Pellizzari

First published in London, United Kingdom, 2023 by IntechOpen
IntechOpen is the global imprint of INTECHOPEN LIMITED, registered in England and Wales, registration number: 11086078, 5 Princes Gate Court, London, SW7 2QJ, United Kingdom

British Library Cataloguing-in-Publication Data
A catalogue record for this book is available from the British Library

Additional hard and PDF copies can be obtained from orders@intechopen.com

Controversies in Liver Transplantation - Recent Challenges and Future Perspectives
Edited by Dipesh Kumar Yadav
p. cm.
Print ISBN 978-1-80356-071-7
Online ISBN 978-1-80356-072-4
eBook (PDF) ISBN 978-1-80356-073-1

Meet the editor

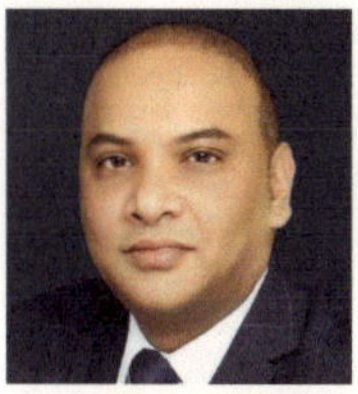

Dr. Dipesh Kumar Yadav received an MBBS from Taishan Medical University, China, and an MD in General Surgery from Ningbo University, China. He obtained a Ph.D. and postdoc in Hepatobiliary Surgery and Liver Transplantation from the School of Medicine, Zhejiang University, China. In 2019, he won the Postdoctoral Exchange Fellowship Program (Talent Introduction Program) from the Postdoctoral Foundation of China. Dr. Yadav has published numerous articles in high-impact journals. He is an experienced surgeon in open/laparoscopic hepatobiliary and pancreatic surgery, including liver transplantation, the Whipple procedure, hepatectomy, laparoscopic pancreaticoduodenectomy, pancreas distal resection, and so on. His research interests include liver transplantation, intestine transplantation, liver cancer, pancreatic cancer, hepatobiliary and pancreatic surgery, transplant oncology, and transplant immunology.

Contents

Preface

This book examines controversial issues in the field of liver transplantation. The chapters are evidence-based and discuss liver transplantation for acute or chronic liver failure, liver transplantation for alcoholic liver disease, and economic considerations of liver transplantation. This volume is a useful resource for hepatologists, liver transplant surgeons, medical residents, medical students, and others interested in transplant surgery.

We would like to thank IntechOpen for giving us an opportunity to publish this book.

Dr. Dipesh Kumar Yadav, MBBS, MD, Ph.D., Postdoc
The First Affiliated Hospital of Zhejiang University,
Hangzhou, China

Chapter 1

Introductory Chapter: Liver Transplant in the Current Era

Dipesh Kumar Yadav, Rajesh Kumar Yadav and Tingbo Liang

1. Introduction

The historical backdrop of liver transplantation (LT) is an intricate story to reveal. It is an adventure of extraordinary achievement and catastrophic disappointments. Throughout the history of LT, controversies and LT seem to be synonymous with each other.

To begin with the world's first liver transplant, which was done by Thomas Starzl on March 1963 in a 3-years-old boy with biliary atresia, and another five more LT were performed by Thomas Starzl in the following years, but none of them survived more than 23 days [1]. During that time, many called a liver transplant as an unethical procedure and condemned Starzl. After the discovery of cyclosporine A, the survival of LT patients significantly increased [2, 3]. Additionally, in recent years, the advancement in surgical techniques, new antimicrobials and immunosuppressant drugs, and cutting-edge interventional radiology have notably enhanced the outcomes of LT. At present, LT turned out to be the gold standard and only the cure for end-stage liver diseases. The outcomes of LT recipients have significantly enhanced throughout the years through therapeutic advances, including ameliorated surgical techniques, powerful antimicrobial treatment, effective immunosuppressive drug regimens, and cutting-edge interventional radiology. At present, LT turned out to be the gold standard and only the cure for end-stage liver diseases. Despite the improvements in results, LT is still facing lots of challenges, where demand is high and the resources, primarily concerned with donors, are very limited. Although the marginal supply of organ donors has been increased through different surgical and medical innovations [4, 5]. Nonetheless, there are many unsolved questions that need in-depth debate among the transplant society, primarily focusing on the question about the selection of patients that are in need of LT, best use of new drugs, and procedures in this area, which has quickly advanced in the course of recent decades [4–7]. It is believed that DCD-LT poses higher risks of graft failure and biliary complication in comparison with donation after brain death (DBD) LT, which are related to warm ischemia, early allograft dysfunction, and prolonged cold ischemia time [5]. Similarly, in the time of organ shortage, the strategy of salvage liver transplant (SLT) is used for patients with HCC in the case of recurrence after resection [6]. However, SLT still remains controversial in comparison to primary liver transplant (PLT) mainly due to surgical difficulties due to adhesions, increased rate of posttransplant complications, and poor long-term outcomes [6]. Likewise, the approach of ABOi LT was to increase the donor pool and to provide LT in emergency conditions. However, ABOi LT remains to be a controversial approach in comparison to ABO-compatible (ABOc) LT, mainly due to different risks associated with it, especially earlier graft loss, acute cellular rejection (ACR), antibody-mediated rejection (AMR), vascular, biliary complications, and HCC recurrence [4]. Moreover, other concerns are related to timing, economic evaluations, and criteria of LT for acute decompensated liver and LT for severe alcoholic hepatitis as tools for decision-making and implications in clinical practice [8–10].

To review all the contentions in LT comprehensively is outside the sphere of this chapter. This chapter is principally aims at LT for Hepatitis C virus (HCV)-related cirrhosis and nutritional support for cachectic patients waiting for LT.

2. Liver transplant and hepatitis C virus (HCV)

Hepatitis C virus (HCV) infection accounts for approximately around 40% of all chronic liver diseases in the United States [11]. However, since the introduction of direct-acting antiviral (DAA) therapy, the number of cases has declined rapidly in recent years. Nonetheless, HCV-related cirrhosis is still the third most common indication for LT in the United States [12]. It is recommended that all the patients with HCV infection should be treated ahead of LT. If not treated in the pretransplant setup, there is a very high chance of HCV reinfection after liver transplant, and that can be the main cause of graft failure without effective antiviral therapy [13].

It is unclear if the HCV-positive patients with child grade C on the LT waiting list should be treated with antiviral drugs before liver transplant. It is seen that the practice varies largely in different regions and medical centers.

The primary consideration is the accessibility and utilization of HCV-positive livers. In regions where these organs are extremely common, the accentuation will probably be not to treat HCV-infected patients who are on the LT waiting list with the goal that HCV-positive livers can be available for such patients. Similarly, in the regions where HCV-positive livers are not as common, the focus will be toward treating HCV-positive patients before the LT. A recent study by Bowring et al., showed large variations in the centers using HCV-positive liver, which ranges between 0 and 40%. Indeed, roughly one-fourth of the medical centers by no means have used an HCV-positive liver, while at one medical center 40% of liver from HCV-infected donors were used [14]. Accordingly, there is a vast disparity in the utilization of HCV-positive livers. The choice to treat patients before the LT is situated to some extent on this issue.

Besides, the model for end-stage liver disease (MELD) score, before LT is an additional circumstance from above. In an HCV-positive patient with a low MELD score, physicians focus on treating such patients with DDA prior to transplant, which can make them virus-free with a sustained virologic response (SVR). However, in the patients whose MELD scores are more than 30, physicians are less likely to treat those patients with DDA prior to LT and place them in a situation called "MELD limbo" or "MELD purgatory." Saying that refers to the patients who are not too sick to undergo LT, yet not in a good health to function satisfactorily. This has extensively been debated concerning why patients ought not to be treated [15].

The last reason to acknowledge is the patient's capacity for *medication* adherence and completing the course of the DDA, which is normally 12 weeks. Most patients with decompensated liver fail to complete their course due to repeated hospitalization. Likewise, it has been found that the patients with decompensated liver have a lower SVR rate contrasted with less sick patients [16].

Despite, it is hard to generalize the treatment strategies of different centuries, overall most of the centers might say that patients with MELD scores of 20 or above are likely not great candidates for HCV antiviral treatment. Whatever the reason, this practice greatly varies from hospital to hospital and geographical location, which depends on the physician's judgment, the availability of HCV-positive organs, and the MELD score of patients before LT.

3. Nutritional support for cachectic patients before liver transplant

Currently, frailty, and sarcopenia are have gained lots of concern in LT, as they have shown to *associated with* an increased risk of morbidity and mortality for the patient waiting for LT and post-LT [17, 18]. Frailty is evaluated through different performance-based parameters, such as grasp strength and gait speed, chair stands, and balance [19], whereas sarcopenia is regularly evaluated by estimating the psoas muscle zone on imaging or using whole-body bioelectrical impedance [20]. Nonetheless, presently there are many ongoing studies to properly identify these patients and appraise them for new treatments [18].

High mortality has been reported in the patients on the waiting list who are malnourished, and those on a low protein diet of less than 0.8 gm/kg body weight/ day [21]. In a study by Le Cornu et al., found that nutritional advice together with oral nutritional supplements improved the mid-arm circumference and grasp strength of the patients compared to nutritional advice alone; nonetheless, mortality was similar in both groups [22]. Similarly, a pilot study by Plank et al., revealed that oral nutritional supplements fortified with omega-3 fatty acids, arginine, and nucleotides had lower infectious complications after LT than those on the standard nutritional intervention [23]. However, a successive randomized trial by Plank et al., did not find any significant benefits of perioperative immunonutrition in patients undergoing LT in terms of preoperative nutritional status or postoperative outcome compared to standard oral nutritional intervention [24]. Similarly, a meta-analysis found that perioperative use of immunonutrition, such as glutamine or omega-3 fatty acids, arginine, and ribonucleic acids, was significantly associated with a reduction in infectious complications and earlier recovery in liver function after LT; however, there was no significant difference in overall survival [25]. Kaido et al., also reported that patients who took oral immunonutrition, has less postoperative infectious complications after LT [26]. Surprisingly, preoperative branched-chain amino acid only showed better survival outcomes for patients with sarcopenic on the waiting list; however, it failed to improve survival in non-sarcopenic patients.

The molecular mechanisms of integral sarcopenia have been researched extensively and interpreted to some degree. In the meantime, a unique idea has developed, for example, the incidence of overweight and corpulence in cirrhotic patients [27]. This warrants both clinical consideration and further investigation. Lately, studies have provided initial information on the potential advantage of physical activity in cirrhotic patients [28–30]. However, these data need to be better defined and verified.

To conclude, liver glycogen is exhausted in patients with cirrhosis. Thus, it is prudent to take incredible consideration to minimize the interval without nutrient consumption, so as to dodge gluconeogenesis from muscle protein in previously protein-depleted patients. The interest to characterize and treat frailty and sarcopenia in patients waiting for LT is rapidly increasing. In spite of the fact that results from the studies cited above are encouraging, there is a lack of large, well-powered homogeneous groups of patients, and long-term observational studies that can provide the ideal treatment for anticipation or reversal of frailty and sarcopenia.

4. Future perspectives

In general, LT is an exhilarating field of research. It comprises with an opportunity a wide range of research areas, such as transplant immunology, transplant pharmacology, transplant oncology, infectious diseases, and cardiovascular diseases.

Author details

Dipesh Kumar Yadav[1,2,3,4,5]*, Rajesh Kumar Yadav[6] and Tingbo Liang[1,2,3,4,5]

1 Department of Hepatobiliary Surgery and Pancreatic Surgery, The First Affiliated Hospital, Zhejiang University, Hangzhou, China

2 Zhejiang Provincial Key Laboratory of Pancreatic Disease, The First Affiliated Hospital, Zhejiang University, Hangzhou, China

3 Zhejiang Provincial Innovation Center for the Study of Pancreatic Diseases, The First Affiliated Hospital, Zhejiang University, Hangzhou, China

4 Zhejiang Provincial Clinical Research Center for the Study of Hepatobiliary and Pancreatic Diseases, The First Affiliated Hospital, Zhejiang University, Hangzhou, China

5 Cancer Center, Zhejiang University, Zhejiang, China

6 Department of Clinical Pharmacology, University of Louisiana at Monroe, Monroe, LA, United States

*Address all correspondence to: 2338507593@qq.com

References

[1] Starzl TE, Marchioro TL, Vonkaulla KN, et al. HOMOTRANSPLANTATION OF THE LIVER IN HUMANS. Surgery, Gynecology & Obstetrics. 1963;**117**:659-676

[2] Calne RY, Rolles K, White DJ, et al. Cyclosporin a initially as the only immunosuppressant in 34 recipients of cadaveric organs: 32 kidneys, 2 pancreases, and 2 livers. Lancet. 1979;**2**:1033-1036

[3] Starzl TE, Todo S, Tzakis AG, et al. Liver transplantation: An unfinished product. Transplantation Proceedings. 1989;**21**:2197-2200

[4] Yadav DK, Hua YF, Bai X, et al. ABO-incompatible adult living donor liver transplantation in the era of rituximab: A systematic review and meta-analysis. Gastroenterology Research and Practice. 2019;**2019**:8589402

[5] Chen W, Yadav DK. Liver transplantation from voluntary organ donor system in China: A comparison between DBD and DCD liver transplants. Gastroenterology Research and Practice. 2019;**2019**:5736702

[6] Yadav DK, Chen W, Bai X, et al. Salvage liver transplant versus primary liver transplant for patients with hepatocellular carcinoma. Annals of Transplantation. 2018;**23**:524-545

[7] Yadav DK, Adhikari VP, Ling Q, et al. Immunosuppressants in liver transplant recipients with coronavirus disease 2019: Capability or catastrophe?-a systematic review and meta-analysis. Frontiers in Medicine (Lausanne). 2021;**8**:756922

[8] Yadav DK, Yadav RK, Liang T. Acute decompensated liver: When to transplant? In: Yadav DK, editor. Controversies in Liver Transplantation - Recent Challenges and Future Perspectives [Working Title] [Internet]. London: IntechOpen; 2022 [cited 2022 Oct 11]. Available from: https://www.intechopen.com/online-first/82100. DOI: 10.5772/intechopen.105350

[9] Yadav DK, Zhang Q, Bai X, et al. Liver transplantation for alcohol-related liver disease (ARLD): An update on controversies and considerations. Canadian Journal of Gastroenterology and Hepatology. 2020;**2020**:8862152

[10] Villafuerte SR, Veríssimo AR, Mochas LG, Zurita FA, Salazar JP. Economic evaluations of liver transplantation as tools for decision-making and implications in clinical practice. In: Yadav DK, editor. Controversies in Liver Transplantation - Recent Challenges and Future Perspectives [Working Title] [Internet]. London: IntechOpen; 2022 [cited 2022 Oct 11]. Available from: https://www.intechopen.com/online-first/81869. DOI: 10.5772/intechopen.104903

[11] Younossi ZM, Birerdinc A, Henry L. Hepatitis C infection: A multi-faceted systemic disease with clinical, patient reported and economic consequences. Journal of Hepatology. 2016;**65**:S109-s119

[12] Chedid MF. Nonalcoholic steatohepatitis: The second leading indication for liver transplantation in the USA. Digestive Diseases and Sciences. 2017;**62**:2621-2622

[13] Grassi A, Ballardini G. Post-liver transplant hepatitis C virus recurrence: An unresolved thorny problem. World Journal of Gastroenterology. 2014;**20**:11095-11115

[14] Bowring MG, Kucirka LM, Massie AB, et al. Changes in utilization and discard of hepatitis C-infected donor livers in the recent era. American Journal of Transplantation : Official Journal of the American Society of Transplantation and the American Society of Transplant Surgeons. 2017;**17**:519-527

[15] Carrion AF, Khaderi SA, Sussman NL. Model for end-stage liver disease limbo, model for end-stage liver disease purgatory, and the dilemma of treating hepatitis C in patients awaiting liver transplantation. Liver Transplantation. 2016;**22**:279-280

[16] Ohkoshi S, Hirono H, Yamagiwa S. Direct antiviral agent treatment of decompensated hepatitis C virus-induced liver cirrhosis. World Journal of Gastrointestinal Pharmacology and Therapeutics. 2015;**6**:114-119

[17] Kaido T, Ogawa K, Fujimoto Y, et al. Impact of sarcopenia on survival in patients undergoing living donor liver transplantation. American Journal of Transplantation. 2013;**13**:1549-1556

[18] Merli M, Berzigotti A, Zelber-Sagi S, et al. EASL clinical practice guidelines on nutrition in chronic liver disease. Journal of Hepatology. 2019;**70**:172-193

[19] Lai JC. Editorial: Advancing adoption of frailty to improve the Care of Patients with cirrhosis: Time for a consensus on a frailty index. The American Journal of Gastroenterology. 2016;**111**:1776-1777

[20] Chen H-W, Dunn MA. Arresting frailty and sarcopenia in cirrhosis: Future prospects. Clinical Liver Disease. 2018;**11**:52-57

[21] Englesbe MJ, Patel SP, He K, et al. Sarcopenia and mortality after liver transplantation. Journal of the American College of Surgeons. 2010;**211**:271-278

[22] Le Cornu KA, McKiernan FJ, Kapadia SA, et al. A prospective randomized study of preoperative nutritional supplementation in patients awaiting elective orthotopic liver transplantation. Transplantation. 2000;**69**:1364-1369

[23] Plank LD, McCall JL, Gane EJ, et al. Pre- and postoperative immunonutrition in patients undergoing liver transplantation: A pilot study of safety and efficacy. Clinical Nutrition. 2005;**24**:288-296

[24] Plank LD, Mathur S, Gane EJ, et al. Perioperative immunonutrition in patients undergoing liver transplantation: A randomized double-blind trial. Hepatology. 2015;**61**:639-647

[25] Lei Q, Wang X, Zheng H, et al. Peri-operative immunonutrition in patients undergoing liver transplantation: A meta-analysis of randomized controlled trials. Asia Pacific Journal of Clinical Nutrition. 2015;**24**:583-590

[26] Kaido T, Mori A, Ogura Y, et al. Impact of enteral nutrition using a new immuno-modulating diet after liver transplantation. Hepato-Gastroenterology. 2010;**57**:1522-1525

[27] Montano-Loza AJ, Angulo P, Meza-Junco J, et al. Sarcopenic obesity and myosteatosis are associated with higher mortality in patients with cirrhosis. Journal of Cachexia, Sarcopenia and Muscle. 2016;**7**:126-135

[28] Baar K. Training for endurance and strength: Lessons from cell signaling. Medicine and Science in Sports and Exercise. 2006;**38**:1939-1944

[29] Dietrich R, Bachmann C, Lauterburg BH. Exercise-induced hyperammonemia in patients with compensated chronic liver

disease. Scandinavian Journal of Gastroenterology. 1990;**25**:329-334

[30] Berzigotti A, Albillos A, Villanueva C, et al. Effects of an intensive lifestyle intervention program on portal hypertension in patients with cirrhosis and obesity: The SportDiet study. Hepatology. 2017;**65**:1293-1305

Chapter 2

Economic Evaluations of Liver Transplantation as Tools for Decision-Making and Implications in Clinical Practice

Santiago Rodríguez Villafuerte, Adilson Renato Veríssimo, Luis Geovanny Mochas, Fabian Andrés Zurita and Julio Patricio Salazar

Abstract

The economic theory of liver transplant (LT) and issues specifically related to the waiting list are still in their early days, not being fully explored from the theoretical, empirical point of view and their implications for the formulation of evidence-based public policies. The success of each LT stage (pre-LT, LT, and post-LT) is based on the success of the previous one, hence the need for a detailed study of each of them. Previous economic analyses have focused only on the cost of LT. However, comprehensive economic assessments that allow the integrated and detailed study of each of the steps will allow investment in the most critical points of the processes. In this way, there will be effective management with the elaboration and implementation of public policies that make processes more cost-effective, maximizing the benefit of LT. Our chapter will focus on the pharmacoeconomic study of the different stages that make up LT in chronic liver diseases. It will also allow reflection and analysis of the policies established in transplant centers; in this way to make better use of resources and seek a greater benefit from the transplant.

Keywords: liver transplant, economic evaluation, public policies, cirrhosis, portal hypertensión

1. Introduction

In recent decades, epidemiological changes and technological advances warned in the health sector have improved the quality of life of patients and reduced the morbidity and mortality rates of a significant number of diseases [1–3].

The wide range of health technologies—medicines, materials, equipment, procedures, organizational, educational, information, and support systems that allow health care and care—have made it necessary to analyze evidence-based analysis, taking into account aspects such as efficacy, accuracy, effectiveness, and costs in the decision-making process, so that they can be made available in health systems; consequently, there is a constant concern with the sustainability of health systems and the ability to maintain long-term benefits, thus in order to evaluate the relationship between the health sector budget and the different technologies, economic assessments emerged, since the different interventions compete with each other for finite resources—cumulative technologies, non-substitute [1–4].

Among the technologies (procedures) that have improved in the last six decades is solid organ transplantation, which evolved from experimental procedures to standard procedures that save lives [5].

Regarding the area of hepatology and liver transplantation (LT), the first economic evaluations date back to the 1990s and described only the cost of LT [6–8]. Further analyses focused on the economic impact of different liver diseases [9–13] and on cost-effectiveness and cost-utility studies of treatments and screening tools for both liver diseases and their decompensation [14–19].

However, data on costs related to the management of patients on the waiting list and the economic impact of complications of chronic liver disease in this clinical scenario as well as in the follow-up of patients in the post-LT are scarce and should be considered in the global evaluation [20–23]; in this sense, this chapter seeks to contribute to: (a) debate, (b) decision-making process, and (c) development of evidence-based public policies that allow maximizing the benefit of LT in chronic liver diseases and minimizing the cost of opportunity in a scenario with limited resources.

We will also carry out a short review of pharmacoeconomic studies in the scenario of LT in acute liver failure.

2. General concepts

LT is the therapeutic option of choice for patients with acute or chronic end-stage liver failure (**Table 1**) [24–26]. It should be recommended for patients whose estimated survival after LT exceeds or exceeds life expectancy without the procedure or when it is expected to enable significant improvement in quality of life [27].

The survival benefit is considerable. In Europe, according to the European Liver Transplant Registry (ELTR), survival rates in 1 and 5 years are 83 and 71%, respectively [28].

In the United States, according to the Organ Procurement and Transplantation Network (OPTN)/United Network for Organ Sharing (UNOS), survival rates for recipients who received deceased donor grafts are 91.2% in the first year and 75% in the fifth year [29].

Cirrhosis, by any etiology, is the most frequent indication of LT [30, 31]; however, the diagnosis of cirrhosis per se does not justify the indication of LT. Although cirrhotic patients have lower survival when compared with the general population, the presence of decompensation of the underlying liver disease does not completely justify the indication, even because many of them can be controlled or avoided with effective medical treatments [31, 32].

Patients should be carefully evaluated and prioritized using prognostic models that incorporate clinical and laboratory variables, which helps the indication for LT [24, 31].

Status * OPTN/UNOS		Status II** OPTN/UNOS	
Acute liver failure	Paracetamol poisoning	Chronic liver diseases	Alcoholic liver disease
	Drug-induced liver failure		Nonalcoholic fatty liver disease
	Wilson's disease or Budd-Chiari syndrome		Chronic viral hepatitis
	Nonfunctioning primary graft		Autoimmune liver diseases
	Hepatic artery thrombosis	Other syndromes	Cystic fibrosis
			Familial amyloidotic polyneuropathy
			Primary hyperoxaluria

Table 1.
Indications for enrolling patients on the waiting list.

Currently, in many countries, the severity and risk of death from chronic liver disease are estimated by the MELD score (Model of End-stage Liver Disease), a robust predictor of survival in 3 months [33–35]. For its calculation, three laboratory tests are used: total bilirubin, creatinine, and international normalized ratio (INR) [36].

In other words, the success of the transplant depends, in part, on timely indications, on careful evaluation, on proper prioritization and allocation, and on enough donors. However, when is the appropriate time to indicate The LT and which people should be included in the list are issues that continue to arouse interest and controversy [24, 26, 30].

3. Waiting list management

3.1 Evaluation of candidates and selection

Early identification of patients considered as candidates for LT is crucial to ensure the greatest possible benefit [25–27]. Although the severity of liver disease is the initial concern, a number of considerations guide the evaluation process. Examinations and consultancies preferably performed in the outpatient setting allow: (a) to confirm the lack of effective therapeutic options for underlying liver disease; (b) identify and optimize the factors that may affect the survival of candidates after inclusion on the waiting list; (c) identify, evaluate, and determine the impact of comorbidities on post-LT results; (d) fully evaluate psychosocial aspects and educate candidates and their families about the LT process, post-surgical care, and long-term care to exclude absolute and relative contraindications [25, 31].

Commonly, multidisciplinary teams are composed of hepatologists, transplant surgeons, anesthesiologists, psychiatrists, physicians from other specialties, specialist nurses in LT, nutritionists, psychologists, etc. [25, 31].

There are assessments common to all candidates and others that adapt to specific clinical conditions (**Table 2**).

Grafts should be allocated, ideally, to patients with a higher probability of list death and, at the same time, a higher probability of survival after the LT [37, 38]. However, if, on the one hand, the best LT results are achieved when the patient is not

General evaluation	Clinical, epidemiological, social history and complete physical examination
Hepatological evaluation	Confirm diagnosis of underlying liver disease, assess severity and prognosis, and optimize treatment
Cardiological evaluation	Electrocardiogram Echocardiogram with assessment of pulmonary artery pressure and shunt If cardiologic risk factors are present, non-invasive exercise testing Myocardial perfusion scintigraphy or invasive procedures when necessary
Pulmonary assessment	Chest X-ray, pulmonary function tests, arterial blood gas
Surgical evaluation	Identify technical challenges (previous abdominal surgery, portal vein thrombosis, vascular or bile duct abnormalities), donor options, and transplant type
Infectious diseases	Serology for hepatitis A, B, C and D, HIV, EBV immunoglobulin (Ig) G, CMV IgG, VZV IgG/IgM Tuberculosis, VDRL, FTA-ABS Vaccines: measles, mumps, influenza, diphtheria, whooping cough and tetanus
Laboratory tests	ABO blood group and Rh factor, blood count, coagulogram (V-factor, D-dimer, fibrinogen breakdown products), renal function, electrolytes, lipidogram, liver function tests, glucose, iron profile, protein electrophoresis, thyroid hormones, IgA, IgG, IgM, prostate antigen
Imaging exams	Ultrasonography (USG) of the abdomen (Doppler if necessary), computed tomography (CT) or nuclear magnetic resonance (NMR) of the abdomen and thorax, facial mass
Dental/maxillofacial assessment	Identify infectious processes: caries, abscesses, tooth extractions if necessary
Psychiatry	History about alcohol consumption, drugs, psychiatric illnesses. Optimize treatment when needed
Social service	Assess support network, adherence, effect of LTx on the patient's personal and social life, pre and post LTx counseling
Nutritional assessment	Identify factors that may affect the results: malnourished, obese, sarcopenic patients
Specific ratings by sex and age	Gynecological/urological/dermatological evaluation Colonoscopy, endoscopy

Table 2.
Processes in the evaluation period for enrollment in the waiting list.

decompensated and has a good general condition, on the other hand, it is decompensated patients who need urgent LT because they have a worse prognosis [39].

The dissociation between the number of candidates and donors remains one of the greatest limitations for performing transplants. This creates an extremely complex situation in the management of waiting lists [30, 31]. Once the MELD model with good prognostic capacity was defined in terms of short-term survival of cirrhotic patients, we tried to define a cutoff point from which patients should be included in the list. A study [37] conducted in the United States evaluated 12,996 patients included on the waiting list for LT between 2001 and 2003 (patients listed for acute liver failure and hepatocelullar carcinoma (HCC) were excluded from the analysis). Patients were followed up until death on a list or 1-year post-LT. At the time of inclusion, more than 50% of the candidates had <15 points and, at the end of the follow-up period, 24% of the LT were performed in patients with MELD <15. Among the patients who were still on the waiting list, 75.9% of those included in the list with a score between 6 and 11 remained with the same score and less than 5% had a higher score. Regarding death rates in 1 year after the LT, patients who transplanted with <15 scores had 3.66 times [confidence interval (CI): 2.23–5.95; $p < 0.001$] were more likely to die than patients with higher scores, suggesting that the risk of LT in patients with meld score <15 is higher than the benefit [37]. Thus, in the United States, grafts should be offered at the local and regional level primarily for patients with a MELD >15 [40].

The model has limitations, not aforementioned to the severity of some of the complications of chronic liver disease, such as refractory ascites, portosystemic encephalopathy, and HCC. Situations in which the score does not reflect the natural history of the disease are known as special situations. For patients with special situations, points are awarded, independent of the calculated MELD score, which would be equivalent to the increase in mortality while on the waiting list. The score attributed to these patients is different between countries and/or transplant centers.

4. Economic assessments

4.1 On the waiting list

In the United States, the waiting list stay time for LT is approximately 11 months and has been decreasing [41]. Longer list times may mean transplanting patients with more advanced disease and, therefore, less cost-effective transplants, due to increased costs of the procedure and/or pre-LT care [42].

Economic analyses have focused on the economic impact of liver disease and the cost of LT, without considering that waiting list patient management is also a costly process [20–23].

The lack of integrated medical records between outpatient services and hospitalizations and specific software for hospital management, in addition to overhead costs not always available in hospital cost appropriation systems, makes it difficult to study the economic impact of waiting list management [20–22].

The inclusion of patients on the waiting list for the LT comprises two subperiods: (a) evaluation, during which the need for the patient to be transplanted and investigated the presence of absolute or relative contraindications; and (b) permanence in the list, from the date of inclusion to the outcome, be it transplantation, death, or exclusion. However, studies evaluating the cost of waiting list management have focused on the length of stay on the list.

A retrospective North American study [20] evaluated costs of 58 patients included in the waiting list between November 1996 and December 1997. The analysis included different moments: permanence on the waiting list (treatments for liver disease, comorbidities, and complications), perioperative, and post-LT. The costs were grouped into five categories: professional and hospital services during hospitalizations, organ uptake, outpatient services, and post-LT medications. Costs related to outpatient consultations or examinations performed outside the transplant center were not included. After 2.5 years of follow-up, there were 19% of deaths on the waiting list, 36% remained on the waiting list, and 45% had undergone transplantation. While waiting lists, patients had 9.7 outpatient visits and 3.1 hospitalizations (52.8 days/patient or 3062 days in total). The cost associated with hospitalizations was US$ 3.37 million (for every dollar spent on professional services during hospitalizations, an additional amount of US$ 2.75 corresponding to hospital expenses was requested to support the services). The subgroup analysis found that the cost to stay on the waiting list on an average of 14 months was $1.8 million for the 26 patients who received deceased donor graft ($70,000/patient), $0.3 million for patients who remained on the waiting list ($14,000/patient), and $0.8 million for patients who died on the waiting list ($74,000/patient), statistically significant when compared with that of patients on waiting lists ($p < 0.01$). Spending in the waiting list period accounted for 41% of the total expenditure. The sensitivity analysis indicated that the variation of the dollar per diem by ±50% during hospitalizations would modify the cost of staying on a waiting list between 36 and 46%. The authors pointed out some limitations of the study: it was conducted in a single center, and the average cost of treatment could be explained by the inclusion of young patients with less severe liver disease, even though there was no statistically significant difference between the characteristics of the sample. In addition, they stressed the importance of including care costs from other centers to comprehensively assess the impact of the waiting list on the total cost and the need for national studies enabling more accurate subgroup analyses. In other words, they suggest using the social perspective in future studies [20].

A retrospective North American study [21] with OPTN data analyzed the costs of 990 adult patients submitted to LT (94% of deceased donor and 6% living) between March 2002 and August 2007. Patients undergoing double liver and kidney transplantation were included in the analysis. Using the perspective of health plans, the researchers divided expenses into three periods: pre-LT (365 days before LT up to 3 days before admission to LT), LT (2 days before admission to LT up to 90 days post-LT), and post-LT (91–365 days post-LT). Of the 990 patients included in the analysis, 778 had health insurance coverage in the pre-LT, 690 in transplantation, and 678 in the post-LT, and 365 patients had coverage in the three periods. The costs were associated with the MELD score at the time of transplantation. Patients with a MELD score <20 points were more frequently white, presented etiology of HCV liver disease associated with HCV, and received grafts from a living donor ($p < 0.005$). Patients with ≥21 points had more frequent double liver and kidney transplantation, had more frequent liver disease decompensation (ascites and portossystemic encephalopathy), and had time on mechanical ventilation and in the ICU after the greater LT ($p < 0.05$). Regarding the severity of liver disease, the MELD score at the time of LT was significantly associated with pre-LT and post-LT ($p < 0.0001$) costs in the univariate model (MELD 6–14: US$ 77,100 ± 86,800; MELD 15–20: US$ 92,400 ± 110,500; MELD 21–27: $158,300 ± 262,300; MELD 28–40: $237,300 ± 229,800). After adjusting the values for age, diagnosis of HCV, HBV, HCV, ABO group and re-LT, it was observed that patients with MELD score 28–40 points and submitted to double liver and kidney transplantation had statistically higher costs compared with the other groups in the pre-LT and transplantation period (MELD 28–40: US$ 145,500 and US$ 60,700; double transplantation: $178,300 and $90,900, respectively). The authors pointed out that the main driver of the high cost of LT is the pre-LT and LT costs [21].

US researchers [22] using data from OPTN/UNOS and the American Public Health System (Medicare) studied the association between the cost of waiting list stay and the severity of liver disease, assessed by the MELD score. We analyzed 15,710 adult patients of both sexes, included on the waiting list between 2002 and 2008. In both cohorts—OPTN/UNOS and Medicare—the median age was 56.2 and 46.3 years, respectively. The most frequent etiology of liver disease was HCV, and 8% of patients had associated HCC. The most frequent comorbidities were type II diabetes mellitus and hypertension. The monthly cost of patients on the waiting list was $1805. However, medical costs varied according to the MELD score, being higher in those with more severe diseases and, therefore, with higher scores. In patients with a MELD score 5–10, the average expenditure was US$ 260 ± 2453, while in those with a MELD score of 35–40, it was US$ 33,792 ± 118,952. Age (p = 0.01), female gender (p = 0.03), and diagnosis of HCC (p = 0.03) were associated with higher costs during waiting list stay. The increase in the MELD score during the waiting list was associated with higher costs (US$ 165 for each additional MELD point; p < 0.0001), and expenses with more severe patients (with MELD >30) score were 10 times higher compared with less severe patients (MELD <20 points). As warned by the authors, the study presented some limitations: (a) the cohort studied represented only patients with Medicare health insurance, that is, 27% of the population listed for LT during the study period; (b) higher MELD scores were reported more frequently than lower scores, which could lead to underreporting of these patients. On the other hand, the costs reported by Medicare ensured that the differences in expenditure reflected the actual intensity of resource use. The authors also emphasized that cirrhotic patients with less social support may require more additional care and social services, leading to higher costs [22].

A prospective Brazilian study [23] based on the microcosting methodology evaluated the total cost of patients on the waiting list for LT and the costliest resources. Adult patients enrolled on the waiting list for the LT between January 2012 and December 2013 were prospectively followed up until the date of transplantation, death, exclusion or, at the end of the follow-up, if still on the list. For the analysis, the patients were subdivided into four groups (quartiles) according to the severity of the disease, estimated by the MELD score. The data were obtained through the analysis of medical records and included: number of consultations with health professionals, number of tests performed (laboratory or image), number and type of procedures performed, and hospitalizations. When the analysis was performed, of the 482 patients included, 27.8% had been transplanted, 21.4% had been removed from the waiting list, 13.9% had died, and 36.9% remained on the list. The mean number of hospitalizations per patient was 1.4. In the inclusion in the list, 27.39% had ≤ MELD score, 17 points, 25.31% had a MELD score of 18–24 points, 23.44% had a MELD score of 25–30 points, and 23.86% had a MELD score ≥ 30 points. The total cost to attend for 24 months the 492 patients was US$ 6,064,986.51. Of this total, US$ 1,965,045.52 (32.4%) were generated by outpatient services and US$ 4,099,940.99 (67.60%) per hospitalization. In the outpatient setting, the costliest sectors were: medications (44.31%), clinical analyses and imaging tests (31.68%), and medical professionals (8.96%). During hospitalizations, the most onerous sectors were: medications (35.2%), daily in hospitalization units (26.38%), and imaging tests and clinical analyses (16.72%). Regarding the MELD score, the highest costs were for patients with MELD 25–30 (US$ 16,686.74 ± 16,105.02), being lower for patients with MELD <17 (US$ 5703.22 ± 9318.68). The cost was directly proportional to the number of hospitalizations and hospitalization time [23].

4.2 In LT

The first economic assessments of liver transplantation began in 1990 [43–50] in developed countries. The vast majority were retrospective studies that evaluated transplantation for both chronic diseases and acute liver failure. One of them evaluated double liver-kidney transplantation and the other with an inter-living donor. These studies used different and variable methodologies, considering different periods and long follow-up, which is why there is no uniformity of data or an idea of certain costs (**Table 3**).

Author	Gilbert et al.	Showstack et al.	Rufat et al.	Brown et al.	Markman et al.	Agothoven et al.	Filipponi et al.	Trotter et al.
Parents	US	US	France	US	US	Netherlands	Italy	US
Year	1991–1996	1991–1994	1994–1995	1992–1993	1992–1998	1993–1997	1997–2000	1997–2001
Sample (n)	144	711	38	109	1148	100	252	67
Outline	Retrospective	Prospective	Prospective	Retrospective (Tx Conj. Fig. Kidney)	Retrospective	Retrospective	Retrospective	Prospective
Cost elements	Direct costs (from pre-LT to hospital discharge)	Direct costs (from LTx to hospital discharge excluding professional fees)	Direct costs (from pre-TxH to 1 year after Tx)	Direct costs (from LTx to hospital discharge)	Direct costs (from pre-LT to hospital discharge)	Direct costs (from pre-TxH to 1 year after Tx)	Direct costs (from pre-TxH to 1 year after Tx)	Direct costs (from pre-TxH to 1 year after Tx)
Donor type	Deceased donor	Deceased donor	Deceased donor	Deceased donor	Donor deceased	Donor deceased	Deceased donor	Deceased donor and living
Euro costs (€)	132.930 ± 47.079	154,610	86,515	116,866	Not reported	107,675—for chronic liver disease, and 90,192—for acute liver insuf	75.747 ± 83.846	102.220 ± 123,600
Risk factors for high cost	Not reported	Donor and recipient age Retransplant	Retransplantation, advanced age (>40 years), Grav. of liver disease, Rej. sharp	Pre -Tx kidney function Insuff—fulminant liver disease (UNOS Status I)	Pre Renal Tx Mechanical ventilation dependent	Not reported	Pre Renal Tx non-alcoholic liver disease insuf hep Fulm, Portal vein thrombosis	Not reported

Table 3.
LTx economic assessments.

Due to the development and improvement of more objective mathematical models, which took into account selected risk factors for chronic liver disease and the subsequent adoption of the MELD score for organ allocation, previous research aimed to evaluate the economic burden of liver transplantation according to MELD-based levels of liver disease severity.

Willians et al. [51] determined that the average value of liver transplantation in Memphis, United States, was $92,866 in 1984 (the value updated by inflation for 1995 is approximately $150,000), ranging from $34,997 to 319,337.

Researchers from Turkey in 2011 [52] evaluated the costs of liver transplantation from the admission of pre-transplant to hospital discharge from 1999 to 2009. The sample consisted of 279 patients, the mean age of the recipients was 35.7 ± 14.1 years, and 70.6% were men. The main etiology of transplantation was HBV (44.8% n = 125), HCV (12.5% n = 35), alcoholic liver disease (6.5% n = 18), cryptogenic cirrhosis (7.9% n = 22). One-hundred and eighty-four (184) patients (65.9%) had MELD from 11 to 20; seven patients (2.5%) had MELD around 31 points, with a correlation to CTP 53.8% (n = 150), belonged to class B, and 38.8% (n = 108) belonged to class C. The average length of hospital stay was 39.4 days in 1999 and 41.7 days for 2009. There was no significant difference when comparing the length of hospital stay with body mass index, MELD, and CTP scores.

The researchers concluded that the medical items that generated the highest costs during the study period were medications, medical equipment, and the operating room. There was no statistically significant difference between the etiology of transplantation and cost [52].

When compared with the MELD score, there was no significant MELD difference between 1 and 10 (n = 45) US$ 28,539; MELD between 11 and 20 (n = 184) US$ 30,798; MELD between 21 and 30 (n = 43) US$ 32,564; MELD ≥31 (n = 7) $35,478. Regarding CTP, there was a significant difference with $p < 0.01$ CTP A (n = 21), spent US$ 34,664; CTP B (n = 150) US$ 27,821; CTP C (n = 108) US$ 34,245.

The researchers also concluded that the transplant, when performed in a living donor, presented higher costs; when compared with deceased donor, $33,454 $27,582, respectively with $p < 0.05$ [52].

The group of Boerr et al. [53] evaluated the cost of LT from the perspective of a high complexity hospital and its relationship with the degree of severity of the underlying liver disease using the MELD score, using microcosting analysis.

The economic analysis included the cost of hospitalization in different areas, cost resulting from diagnostic and therapeutic procedures, as well as payroll. Administrative costs were not assessed. Patients diagnosed with HCC were not included in the analysis because they were transplanted earlier by the additional points in the MELD score.

The authors evaluated 77 patients submitted to LT from 2006 to 2010 and divided them into two groups according to MELD score: group1: MELD score from 6 to 19; group 2: MELD score from 20 to 40. The mean age was 53 ± 14 years, the mean hospitalization was 11.6 ± 8.9 days. The average cost of LT was US$ 33,461 ± 12,896 per patient [53].

The authors concluded that the cost of LT is directly proportional to the MELD score, and the higher the score at the time of transplantation, the higher the cost. (group 1: US$ 30,493 ± 8825 per patient, group 2: US$ 36,506 ± 15,833 per patient with $p = 0.04$). The cost of intensive care unit admission was also related to the MELD score (group 1: US$ 3094 and group 2: US$ 4255 $p = <0.01$) [53].

4.3 In the post-LT

The LT has become one of the main treatments for properly selected patients. Nowadays, the long-term survival has improved, many are being tending outside a post-transplant center, which had led to a general familiarity with the complications that could be presented [54].

Many post-transplant complications are being mentioned in medical literature, listing the most common ones below [55]:

- Acute or chronic rejection.
- Complication of the immunosuppression that includes hypertension, renal failure, malignancy, a variety of dermatological complications, and metabolic diseases such as diabetes mellitus, obesity, hyperlipidemia, and osseous disease.
- Biliary complications.
- Reappearance of primary hepatic disease.
- Thrombosis.

4.3.1 Factors involved in the cost of post-LT

If we consider the economic inversions we make in the pre-transplant and transplant, by itself they generate considerable expenses in the health budget, the post-transplant period, and we are not exclusively talking about the immediate recovery but also about all the treatments and possible complications that could appear in long term; this also ends up influencing the health cost elevations that intervene in this type of processes, not only under the perspective of health systems but also from the people, their families, and/or caregivers.

The post complications of LT are relatively common and expensive. As an example, the acute rejection can be presented with an incidence from 20 to 60%. The infections affect up to 70% of the receptors. The thrombosis of the hepatic artery complicates from 4 to 12% of the liver transplants in adults, and the biliary complications occur with an incidence from 10 to 30%; nevertheless, the incremental costs of them are unknown as well as who will assume the price for the complications (the center or the payer) [56].

Several studies suggest that the post-surgery complications are expensive for both the medic center and the payer. Some data alludes that, from these two, the payers are the ones to endure the highest financial burden associated with the posterior complications, and the average hospital costs can increase more than six times when a complication is presented [57].

The shift of this costs depends of various factors, one of them being the type of complications developed by the patient. In such way, we can observe that the biliary complications and the ones that require a reoperation are associated with an increase of prices [56].

Axelrod et al. [58] mention in their study that in centers found in the highest quartile of complications, the biliary issues significantly associate with more heavy costs compared with the centers in the lowest quartile of complications [58]. It is also known that, in this latter centers, there is a 2.73 times more risk of post-transplant readmission [59].

It has also been observed that even when estimating costs in patients with "ideal" LT, meaning they have no risk of complications, whose post-surgery process results are simple (hospital stay <14 days and home discharge), there still exists a significant variety in the use of resources and the medical attention expenses, so understanding the factors that determine this variability in the costs is vital for diminishing unnecessary outlays [60].

But not only are complications considered a factor in the rise of the post-transplant costs, it is also important to mention that these complications depend on risk factors that existed previously in the transplant, in such way that is mentioned in several studies that diabetes and the dialysis dependency could be considered factors that condition the appearance of subsequent complications; therefore, the increase of the costs [59].

Another factor involved in the variation of the costs is the MELD score. MELD is a system of score that allows us to measure the severity of the chronic liver disease, being able to find that at a higher score in this scale, there will exist a higher financial expense, in which the incomes of the transplant center will not be enough to supply what it's within the process and the recovery, which reflects in an unfortunate way with a financial disincentive for performing transplants on high MELD receptors [56].

Several studies demonstrate that patients that have developed an illness with an extreme severity and have a high MELD score are considered of high cost. In the same way and in relation with the functional state and physical capability, those extremely dependent patients were also classified as high cost. This is supported because, in the pre-surgical and post-surgical results, as the medium of LOHS (Length of Hospital Stay), the duration in ICU (Intensive Care Unit), and the readmission rates in 30 days were slightly elevated for patients of high cost. In that way, it's recommended that, if there exists an improvement in the pre-surgical results of patients with liver transplant with a high MELD score and a physical capacity severely damaged, no further use of costs and resources would be required. With this, post-surgical costs would be reduced [59, 61].

In relation with this MELD score, it has also been seen that the sickest patients, with MELD scores superior to 28, have a survival similar to patients transplanted with a low MELD, and once, out of the immediate post-transplant period, the costs have no difference between high and low MELD scores, mostly explained not only by the success of the transplant but for the costs avoided by the recovery of the patients of their serious diseases [60].

The cost factors in any other type of surgical procedure, especially in general and vascular surgery, are determined by the pre-surgical risk factors of the patient and not by the post-surgical complications, while, in the liver transplant, the pre-surgical factors impulse the costs, but in the post-surgery, the complications are the principal generators of costs [56].

We can also add that the complications of the liver transplant not only represent by themselves an additional cost, but also because they show an increment in the cost of the care associated with them. Because of this, even a short stay does not mean lower costs if there is a complication [60].

It's important to mention that medical literature indicates that the difference in costs is not affected by the quality of the supplier of the treatment, but that the characteristics of the health system do influence as one of the most important explanations of the differences in costs of the liver transplant [57].

The type of graft is also considered another factor to take into account in the post-transplant costs, since the DCD (Donation after Circulatory Death) liver transplants have become more common in the past years, coming to represent up until 17% of all transplants in 2013–2014. However, due to the prolonged warm ischemia time, these allografts are more sensitive to severe reperfusion injuries than DBD (Donation after Brain Stem Death) liver, which would bring as consequence that the receptors of DCD would frequently show lower results of survival, graft rejection rates, post-transplant complications, and health-related quality of life (HR-QoL). Not only this but also ischemic cholangiopathy (IC) is a particular preoccupation in the receptors of DCD and relates with a higher increment of the morbidity, a reduction of HR-QoL, and generally it requires a new transplant. Not because of what is mentioned above, we may stop pointing out that with a strict selection of organs and with highly capable transplant team, the DCD results can be compared with the DBD patients [62].

Another factor to take into consideration while evaluating the costs of the hepatic post-transplant is the age, when the liver disease is presented at an early age, it determines the functional hepatic deterioration, which forces to search alternative treatments as it is the hepatic transplant.

In an analysis done by Showstack and his workmates, it was demonstrated that there exist other two factors that influence the increment of the prices that are related with the older age of the donor, the older age of the receptor, the alcoholic liver disease, Child-Pugh cirrhosis class C, and that patients previous to the transplant have been hypnotized [7, 63, 64].

Indirectly, it is also mentioned in the bibliography that an allograft of a high risk index from the donor, the post-transplant discharge to a rehabilitation center, the hepatic disease by itself plus the preparations for the transplant could weaken the patient, putting them in a low nutritional and immunological state. This could lead to a higher risk of posterior hospitalization after the transplant, with which the post-transplant costs would increment [60].

4.3.2 Some numbers of the post-LT costs

There is no existent data that show the exact post-transplant costs, factors have been mentioned that can influence the increment of this expenses, as well as the causes of why it can increase the costs.

An analysis done by a study mentions that at after 90 days of the hepatic transplant, the economic re-entry supposed 43.785 dollars of extra costs in comparison with the patients that did not re-enter so that the readmissions are associated with the variation of the center and a better utilization of resources [59].

The database of the American University Health System Consortium facilitates the financial data on the economic impact of the hospitalization re-entries for hepatic transplant for every hospitalization registered, mentioning that the average price of the index hospitalization for transplant can be $121,161 (interquartile range (IQR), $94,777–$169,361) besides, the average price associated with the hepatic transplant until 90 days after medical discharge including the admission of the transplant can reach $168,666. The subsequently readmitted patients have elevated prices in their income index ($127,088) in contrast with the patients that were not readmitted ($116,250) [59].

These hospitalization readmissions after the transplant generate a significant economic impact and highlight the obligation to improve the attention at long term in this section of high-risk patients, even more because this data can reflect only one part of the long-term risks associated with chronic immunosuppression, graft rejection, and disease recurrence [59].

Other studies that talk about post-transplant costs mention that the average incremental expense per quality-adjusted life year from the moment in which the patient is included in the donors waiting list up to 27 months after the transplant, especially for primary biliary cholangitis (PBC) patients, alcohol-related liver disease (ARLD), primary sclerosing cholangitis (PSC), is of £29,000 sterling pounds (£1000–£59,000), £48,000 (£12,000–£83,000) and £21,000 (£ 23,000–£ 60,000), respectively. The estimations between cost-effectiveness were lower for patients with ALD during the period of 27 months than for patients with PBC or PSC. In a way, this reflects the costs of the most patients with ALD evaluated for each transplant. Although it is data that not only includes the post-transplant but also suggests an estimation of these expenses [63].

Bonsel et al. published the analysis results of price effectivity of the hepatic transplant done in Netherlands in 1980 in nonalcoholic cirrhotic patients, estimating the costs 2 years from the post-transplant in 226,967 Hfl (approximately £130,000 in actual price). They described that the cost of additional quality-adjusted life year for life was around 51,000 Hfl and 133,000 Hfl (£29,000 and £76,000 in actual prices). Even though these results are transcendental for the practice in United Kingdom, it is probable this cannot be directly generalized with other situations because, as an example, the characteristics of the transplant programs in United Kingdom, United States, and other South American countries are very distinct by the number of transplants done in each country [65].

Also, the costs of the hepatic post-transplant could vary depending on the different immediate complications that could be presented finding in the studies that evidence exists showing that the centers in the higher quartile of biliary complication rates, after the liver transplant, spent $22,895 extra per transplant in comparison to the centers in the lower quartile of complications [58, 60].

According to another study, the increment of the MELD score is also related to higher costs ($4309 per MELD point). It's also related to a reduce in the net income of the transplant center ($1512 per MELD point). It is possible that the contractual reimbursement agreements that are not indexed by disease severity do not reflect the increment in the costs resulting from the MELD system. The increasing severity of the disease, seen with higher MELD scores, is related to attention costs exorbitantly higher for the transplant center. In the generator elements of the incensement of the cost in patients with high MELD scores, we can see higher costs for accommodations and food, as well as an increment in the use of laboratory, radiology, and pharmacy services. All this shows that, apart from existing important increment of the use of necessary resources for treating patients with high MELD scores, the hospital admissions for treating all these necessities could lead to a nonsignificant increase, resulting in a net loss for the transplant center [64].

5. Cost and post-LT survival from acute versus chronic liver disease

Survival rates in post-LT patients for acute liver disease are similar to those in post-LT patients for other indications. This is demonstrated by some studies. Kumar et al. [66] mention that these rates in the patient transplanted for acute liver disease are around 80% at the first year and 75% at 5 years, while Roberts et al. [67] indicate that for patients transplanted for any other cause, these rates are at 85% per year and 74% at 5 years.

Regarding the costs involved in LT for acute liver disease versus another pathology, especially chronic pathology, van Agthoven et al. [68] conducted a study where they compared the costs of these two variables, showed that the economic resources invested in patients for LT for acute disease were € 90,000 while this value amounted to € 107,000 in those with patients with chronic pathology. It is worth mentioning that these costs were estimated up to 1 year post-transplant, it is also important to allude that one of the most important parameters that marked these costs were the days of pre-transplant hospitalization, which can be in the case of chronic pathologies up to 12 days versus 1 or 2 days in acute pathologies [68].

Kumar et al. [66] in their study indicate that some other causes of the increase in these costs may be associated with the development of complications in the immediate postoperative period, with infections being the most common, the development of complications is also associated with the etiology for which the transplant was performed, finding better results in those patients with Wilson's disease versus those who presented acute liver failure due to acetaminophen [66].

Something to consider is that the transplant itself already generates an increase in expenses, since Kumar et al. [66] in their study were able to demonstrate that the costs at days 30, 60, and 365 after a liver transplant versus standard care (that is, in a non-transplanted patient) are 5 times higher, as an example, per year the costs in transplantation were calculated at $ 198,000 against $48,000 in the non-transplanted [66].

6. Conclusion

The LT is the therapeutic option of choice for patients with terminal, acute, or chronic liver diseases, should be recommended when the estimate of survival after LT exceeds or exceeds life expectancy without the procedure or when significantly improves quality of life; however, the selection of candidates should be as judicious as possible, aiming at the best use of resources (for example, grafts) although what is the best use may have different interpretations.

Prioritization using prognostic models allows an adequate allocation due to the limited number of donors. Currently, in many countries, the severity and risk of death from chronic liver disease are estimated by the MELD score; however, the model has limitations, not reflecting with accuracy the severity of some of the complications of chronic liver disease, however, when is the opportune time to indicate The LT and that people should be included in the list are issues that continue to arouse interest and controversies.

The evaluation and waiting list waiting processes for LT are complex and costly, and although the protocols for evaluating and including potential recipients depend solely on each center, there are common problems that should be considered during the decision-making process: (a) disparity between the number of patients on the waiting list and the number of organs available—increases the waiting list length of stay and the morbidity and mortality of potential recipients, with possible waiting list existing for clinical worsening or death, (b) competition among other transplant centers in the same area not only by candidates but also by organs, (c) the epidemiological behavior of chronic liver disease, specific to each area.

About LT and post-LT and considering the different factors that influence the results, it is important to know the costs invested in this way, it is possible to develop and apply strategic decisions aimed at optimizing the available resources and improving the services provided in the pursuit of excellence.

Regarding LT in acute pathologies, the available evidence is scarce, however, by the data exposed would seem to be cost-effective; however we need more evidence to generate conclusions to improve existing policies.

We hope that the evidence presented: (a) contributes to the knowledge of cost management—a fundamental important part for care, in the dimensions of quality and efficiency; (b) allow reflection on the economic analyses of high-cost procedures in the face of the socio-hospital context of health in different countries.

Author details

Santiago Rodríguez Villafuerte[1,2]*, Adilson Renato Veríssimo[3], Luis Geovanny Mochas[4], Fabian Andrés Zurita[5] and Julio Patricio Salazar[5]

1 School of Medicine, Universidade Federal de Ciências da Saúde de Porto Alegre (UFCSPA), Porto Alegre, RS, Brazil

2 Department of Hepatology, Hospital Vozandes Quito—HVQ, Quito, SA, Ecuador

3 Universidade Federal de Juiz de Fora, Juiz de Fora, MG, Brazil

4 Department of Gastroenterology, Hospital General IESS San Francisco, Quito, Ecuador

5 Pontifica Universidad Católica Del Ecuador - Puce, Quito, Ecuador

*Address all correspondence to: santy_rodri03@yahoo.com

References

[1] Araujo DV, Ferraz MB. Impacto econômico do tratamento da cardiopatia isquêmica crônica no Brasil: O desafio da incorporação de novas tecnologias cardiovasculares. Archive of Arquivos Brasileiros de Cardiologia. 2005;**85**(1):1-2

[2] Schramm FR, Escosteguy CC. Bioética e avaliação tecnológica em saúde. Cadernos de Saúde Pública. 2000;**16**(4):951-961

[3] Silva EN, Silva MT, Pereira MG. Health economic evaluation studies: Definition and applicability to health systems and services. Epidemiologia e serviços de saúde (Impresso). 2016;**25**(1):205-207. DOI: 10.5123/S1679-49742016000100023

[4] Gold M, Siegel J, Russel I, Weinstein M. Cost-Effectiveness in Health and Medicine. New York: Oxford University Press; 1996

[5] Keller CA. Solid organ transplantation overview and delection criteria. The American Journal of Managed Care. 2015;**21**(Suppl. 1):S4-S11

[6] Bonsel G, Klompmaker I, Essink-Bot M, Habbema J, Slooff M. Cost-effectiveness analysis of the Dutch liver transplantation programme. Transplantation Proceedings. 1990;**22**:1481-1484

[7] Showstack J, Katz PP, Lake JR, et al. Resource utilization in liver transplantation: Effects of patient characteristics and clinical practice. NIDDK Liver Transplantation Database Group. JAMA. 1999;**281**(15):1381-1386

[8] Evans R, Manninen D, Dong F. An economic analysis of liver transplantation: Costs, insurance coverage, and reimbursement. Gastroenterology Clinics of North America. 1993;**22**:451-473

[9] Rehm J, Samokhvalov AV, Shield KD. Global burden of alcoholic liver diseases. Journal of Hepatology. 2013;**59**(1):160-168. DOI: 10.1016/j.jhep.2013.03.007

[10] Blachier M, Leleu H, Peck-Radosavljevic M, Valla DC, Roudot-Thoraval F. The burden of liver disease in Europe: A review of available epidemiological data. Journal of Hepatology. 2013;**58**(3):593-608. DOI: 10.1016/j.jhep.2012.12.005

[11] Udompap P, Kim D, Kim WR. Current and future burden of chronic nonmalignant liver disease. Clinical Gastroenterology and Hepatology. 2015;**13**(12):2031-2041. DOI: 10.1016/j.cgh.2015.08.015

[12] Peery AF, Crockett SD, Barritt AS, Dellon ES, Eluri S, Gangarosa LM, et al. Burden of gastrointestinal, liver, and pancreatic diseases in the United States. Gastroenterology. Dec 2015;**149**(7):1731-1741.e3. DOI: 10.1053/j.gastro.2015.08.045

[13] Younossi ZM, Blissett D, Blissett R, Henry L, Stepanova M, Younossi Y, et al. The economic and clinical burden of nonalcoholic fatty liver disease in the United States and Europe. Hepatology. 2016;**64**(5):1577-1586. DOI: 10.1002/hep.28785

[14] Cammà C, Cabibbo G, Petta S, Enea M, Iavarone M, Grieco A, et al. Cost-effectiveness of sorafenib treatment in field practice for patients with hepatocellular carcinoma. Hepatology. 2013;**57**(3):1046-1054. DOI: 10.1002/hep.26221

[15] Saab S, Gordon SC, Park H, Sulkowski M, Ahmed A, Younossi Z. Cost-effectiveness analysis of sofosbuvir plus peginterferon/ribavirin in the treatment of chronic hepatitis C virus genotype 1 infection. Alimentary Pharmacology & Therapeutics. 2014;**40**(6):657-675. DOI: 10.1111/apt.12871

[16] Lotfipour AK, Douek M, Shimoga SV, Sayer JW, Han SB, Jutabha R, et al. The cost of screening esophageal varices: Traditional endoscopy versus computed tomography. Journal of Computer Assisted Tomography. 2014;**38**(6):963-967. DOI: 10.1097/RCT.0000000000000147

[17] Leidner AJ, Chesson HW, Xu F, Ward JW, Spradling PR, Holmberg SD. Cost-effectiveness of hepatitis C treatment for patients in early stages of liver disease. Hepatology. 2015;**61**(6):1860-1869. DOI: 10.1002/hep.27736

[18] Tapper EB, Sengupta N, Hunink MG, Afdhal NH, Lai M. Cost-effective evaluation of nonalcoholic fatty liver disease with NAFLD fibrosis score and vibration controlled transient elastography. The American Journal of Gastroenterology. 2015;**110**(9):1298-1304. DOI: 10.1038/ajg.2015.241

[19] Zhang E, Wartelle-Bladou C, Lepanto L, Lachaine J, Cloutier G, Tang A. Cost-utility analysis of nonalcoholic steatohepatitis screening. European Radiology. 2015;**25**(11):3282-3294. DOI: 10.1007/s00330-015-3731-2

[20] Brand DA, Viola D, Rampersaud P, Patrick PA, Rosenthal WS, Wolf DC. Waiting for a liver--hidden costs of the organ shortage. Liver Transplantation. 2004;**10**(8):1001-1010. DOI: 10.1002/lt.20212

[21] Buchanan P, Dzebisashvili N, Lentine KL, Axelrod DA, Schnitzler MA, Salvalaggio PR. Liver transplantation cost in the model for end-stage liver disease era: Looking beyond the transplant admission. Liver Transplantation. 2009;**15**(10):1270-1277. DOI: 10.1002/lt.21802

[22] Axelrod DA, Dzebisashvili N, Lentine K, Segev DL, Dickson R, Tuttle-Newhall E, et al. Assessing variation in the costs of care among patients awaiting liver transplantation. American Journal of Transplantation. 2014;**14**(1):70-78. DOI: 10.1111/ajt.12494

[23] Turri JAO, Decimoni TC, Ferreira LA, Diniz MA, Haddad LBP, Campolina AG. Higher MELD score increases the overall cost on the waiting list for liver transplantation: A micro-costing analysis based study. Arquivos de Gastroenterologia. 2017;**54**(3):238-245. DOI: 10.1590/S0004-2803.201700000-35

[24] Russo FP, Ferrarese A, Zanetto A. Recent advances in understanding and managing liver transplantation. F1000Research. Dec 21 2016;**5**:pii. DOI: 10.12688/f1000research.8768.1

[25] Halliday N, Westbrook RH. Liver transplantation: need, indications, patient selection and pre-transplant care. British Journal of Hospital Medicine (London). May 2 2017;**78**(5):252-259. DOI: 10.12968/hmed.2017.78.5.252

[26] Jackson KR, Cameron A. Liver transplantation: Candidate selection and organ allocation in the United States. International Anesthesiology Clinics. 2017;**55**(2):5-17. DOI: 10.1097/AIA.0000000000000142

[27] Farkas S, Hackl C, Schlitt HJ. Overview of the indications and contraindications for liver transplantation. Cold Spring Harbor Perspectives in Medicine. May 1 2014;**4**(5):pii: a015602. DOI: 10.1101/cshperspect.a015602

[28] European Liver Transplant Registry -ELRT. Evolution of LTs in Europe. [homepage na internet]. Villefuif: European Liver Transplant Registry-ELRT; [acesso em 15 jul 2018]. "Disponível em: http://www.eltr.org/Evolution-of-LTs-in-Europe.html"

[29] Organ Procurement & Transplantation Network. National Data Liver Kaplan-Meir Patient Survival Rates for Transplant Performed: 2008-2015 [homepage na internet]. Richmond, Virginia: Health Resources and Services Administration, U.S. Department of Health & Human Services; [acesso em 16 jul 2018]. "Disponível em: https://optn.transplant.hrsa.gov/data/view-data-reports/national-data/"

[30] European Association for the Study of the Liver. EASL clinical practice guidelines: Liver transplantation. Journal of Hepatology. 2016;**64**(2):433-485. DOI: 10.1016/j.jhep.2015.10.006

[31] Martin P, DiMartini A, Feng S, Brown R Jr, Fallon M. Evaluation for liver transplantation in adults: 2013 practice guideline by the American Association for the Study of Liver Diseases and the American Society of Transplantation. Hepatology. 2014;**59**(3):1144-1165

[32] Fleming KM, Aithal GP, Card TR, West J. All-cause mortality in people with cirrhosis compared with the general population: A population-based cohort study. Liver International. 2012;**32**(1):79-84. DOI: 10.1111/j.1478-3231.2011.02517.x

[33] Said A, Williams J, Holden J, Remington P, Gangnon R, Musat A, et al. Model for end stage liver disease score predicts mortality across a broad spectrum of liver disease. Journal of Hepatology. 2004;**40**(6):897-903. DOI: 10.1016/j.jhep.2004.02.010

[34] Botta F, Giannini E, Romagnoli P, Fasoli A, Malfatti F, Chiarbonello B, et al. MELD scoring system is useful for predicting prognosis in patients with liver cirrhosis and is correlated with residual liver function: A European study. Gut. 2003;**52**(1):134-139

[35] Brandão A, Fuchs SC, Gleisner AL, Marroni C, Zanotelli ML, Cantisani G. Model for the end-stage liver disease and death prediction in a cohort of Brazilian patients on the waiting list for liver transplantation. Clinical Transplantation. 2008;**22**(5):651-656. DOI: 10.1111/j.1399-0012.2008.00860.x

[36] Malinchoc M, Kamath PS, Gordon FD, Peine CJ, Rank J, ter Borg PC. A model to predict poor survival in patients undergoing transjugular intrahepatic portosystemic shunts. Hepatology. 2000;**31**(4):864-871. DOI: 10.1053/he.2000.5852

[37] Merion RM, Schaubel DE, Dykstra DM, et al. The survival benefit of liver transplantation. American Journal of Transplantation. 2005;**5**:307-313. DOI: 10.1111/j.1600-6143.2004.00703.x

[38] Ravaioli M, Grazi GL, Ercolani G, et al. The future challenge in the MELD era: How to match extended-use donors and sick recipients. Transplantation. 2006;**82**(7):987-988. DOI: 10.1097/01.tp.0000238705.29588.fc

[39] D'Amico G, Garcia-Tsao G, Pagliaro L. Natural history and prognostic indicators of survival in cirrhosis: A systematic review of 118 studies. Journal of Hepatology. 2006;**44**(1):217-231. DOI: 10.1016/j.jhep.2005.10.013

[40] Elwir S, Lake J. Current status of iver allocation in the United States. Gastroenterología y Hepatología. 2016;**12**:166-170

[41] Kim WR, Lake JR, Smith JM, Schladt DP, Skeans MA, Harper AM, et al. OPTN/SRTR 2016 annual data report: Liver. American Journal of Transplantation.

2018;**18**(Suppl. 1):172-253. DOI: 10.1111/ajt.14559

[42] Sagmeister M, Müllhaupt B. Is living donor liver transplantation cost-effective? Journal of Hepatology. 2005;**43**(1):27-32. DOI: 10.1016/j.jhep.2005.05.005

[43] Gilbert JR, Pascual M, Schoenfeld DA, Rubin RH, Delmonico FL, Cosimi AB. Evolving trends in liver transplantation: An outcome and charge analysis. Transplantation. 1999;**67**(2):246-253

[44] Showstack J, Katz PP, Lake JR, Brown RS, Dudley RA, Belle S, et al. Resource utilization in liver transplantation: Effects of patient characteristics and clinical practice. NIDDK liver transplantation database group. Journal of the American Medical Association. 1999;**281**(15):1381-1386

[45] Rufat P, Fourquet F, Conti F, Le Gales C, Houssin D, Coste J. Cost and outcomes of liver transplantation in adults: A prospective, 1-year, follow-up study. GRETHECO study group. Transplantation. 1999;**68**(1):76-83

[46] Brown RS Jr, Lake JR, Ascher NL, Emond JC, Roberts JP. Predictors of the cost liver transplantation. Liver Transplantation and Surgery. 1998;**4**(2):170-176

[47] Markmann JF, Markmann JW, Markamann DA, Bacquerizo A, Singer J, Holt CD, et al. Preoperative factors associated with outcome and their impact on resource use in 1148 consecutive primary liver transplants. Transplantation. 2001;**72**(6):1113-1122

[48] van Agthoven M, Metselaar HJ, Tilanus HW, Man RA, IJzermans JN, Martin van Ineveld BM. A comparison if the cost and effects of liver transplantation for acute and for chronic liver failure. Transplant International. 2001;**14**(2):87-94

[49] Filipponi F, Pisati R, Cavicchini G, Ulivieri MI, Ferrara R, Mosca F. Cost and outcome analysis and cost determinants of liver transplantation in a European National Healt Service Hospital. Transplantation. 2003;**75**(10):1731-1736

[50] Trotter JF, Mackenzie S, Wachs M, Bak T, Steinberg T, Polsky P, et al. Comprehensive cost comparison of adult-adult right hepatic lobe living-donor liver transplantation with cadaveric transplantation. Transplantation. 2003;**75**(4):473-476

[51] Williams JW, Vera S, Evans LS. Socioeconomic aspects of hepatic transplantation. The American Journal of Gastroenterology. 1987;**82**(11):1115-1119

[52] Akarsu M, Matur M, Karademir S, Unek T, Astarcioglu I. Cost analysis of liver transplantation in Turkey. Transplantation Proceedings. 2011;**43**(10):3783-3788

[53] Boerr E, Anders M, Mella J, Quiñonez E, Goldaracena N, Orozco F, et al. Cost analysis of liver transplantation in a community hospital: Association with the model for end-stage liver disease, a prognostic index to prioritize the most severe patients. Gastroenterología y Hepatología. 2013;**36**(1):1-6

[54] Magro B, Tacelli M, Mazzola A, Conti F, Celsa C. Biliary complications after liver transplantation: Current perspectives and future strategies. HepatoBiliary Surgery and Nutrition. 2021;**10**(1):76-92. DOI: 10.21037/hbsn.2019.09.01

[55] Boeva I, Karagyozov PI, Tishkov I. Post-liver transplant biliary complications: Current knowledge and therapeutic advances. World Journal of Hepatology. 2021;**13**(1):66-79. DOI: 10.4254/wjh.v13.i1.66

[56] Ammori JB, Pelletier SJ, Lynch R, Cohn J, Ads Y, Campbell DA, et al. Incremental costs of post-liver transplantation complications. Journal of the American College of Surgeons. 2008;**206**(1):89-95. DOI: 10.1016/j.jamcollsurg.2007.06.292

[57] Van Der Hilst CS, IJtsma AJC, Slooff MJH, TenVergert EM. Cost of liver transplantation: A systematic review and meta-analysis comparing the United States with other OECD countries. Medical Care Research and Review. 2009;**66**(1):3-22. DOI: 10.1177/1077558708324299

[58] Axelrod DA, Dzebisashvili N, Lentine KL, Xiao H, Schnitzler M, Tuttle-Newhall JE, et al. Variation in biliary complication rates following liver transplantation: Implications for cost and outcome. American Journal of Transplantation. 2015;**15**(1):170-179. DOI: 10.1111/ajt.12970

[59] Wilson GC, Hoehn RS, Ertel AE, Wima K, Quillin RC 3rd, Hohmann S, et al. Variation by center and economic burden of readmissions after liver transplantation. Liver Transplantation. 2015;**21**(7):953-960. DOI: 10.1002/lt.24112

[60] Dhar VK, Wima K, Kim Y, Hoehn RS, Jung AD, Ertel AE, et al. Cost of achieving equivalent outcomes in sicker patients after liver transplant. HPB: The Official Journal of the International Hepato Pancreato Biliary Association. 2018;**20**(3):268-276. DOI: 10.1016/j.hpb.2017.08.037

[61] Abecassis M. Making dollars and sense out of liver transplantation. Liver Transplant. 2009;**15**(10):1159-1161. DOI: 10.1002/lt.21851

[62] McLean KA, Camilleri-Brennan J, Knight SR, Drake TM, Ots R, Shaw CA, et al. Decision modeling in donation after circulatory death liver transplantation. Liver Transplant. 2017;**23**(5):594-603. DOI: 10.1002/lt.24715

[63] Longworth L, Young T, Buxton MJ, Ratcliffe J, Neuberger J, Burroughs A, et al. Midterm cost-effectiveness of the liver transplantation program of England and Wales for three disease groups. Liver Transplant. 2003;**9**(12):1295-1307. DOI: 10.1016/j.lts.2003.09.012

[64] Axelrod DA, Koffron AJ, Baker T, Al-Saden P, Dixler I, McNatt G, et al. The economic impact of MELD on liver transplant centers. American Journal of Transplantation. 2005;**5**(9):2297-2301. DOI: 10.1111/j.1600-6143.2005.01025.x

[65] Bonsel GJ, van't Veer F, Habbema JDF, Klompmaker IJ, Slooff MJH. Use of prognostic models for assessment of value of liver transplantation in primary biliary cirrhosis. Lancet. 1990;**335**(8688):493-497. DOI: 10.1016/0140-6736(90)90734-M

[66] Kumar R, Anand U, Priyadarshi RN. Liver transplantation in acute liver failure: Dilemmas and challenges. World Journal of Transplantation. 2021;**11**(6):187-202. DOI: 10.5500/wjt.v11.i6.187

[67] Roberts MS, Angus DC, Bryce CL, Valenta Z, Weissfeld L. Survival after liver transplantation in the United States: A disease-specific analysis of the UNOS database. Liver Transplantation. 2004;**10**(7):886-897. DOI: 10.1002/lt.20137

[68] van Agthoven M, Metselaar HJ, Tilanus HW, de Man RA, IJzermans JN. Martin van Ineveld BM. A comparison of the costs and effects of liver transplantation for acute and for chronic liver failure. Transplant International. 2001;**14**(2):87-94. DOI: 10.1007/s001470050852

Chapter 3

Acute Decompensated Liver: When to Transplant?

Dipesh Kumar Yadav, Rajesh Kumar Yadav and Tingbo Liang

Abstract

Currently, liver transplant (LT) is only the effective treatment for an acute decompensated liver. Yet, a result of LT in the background of acute decompensated liver largely depends upon the cause of decompensation. Acute-on-chronic liver failure (ACLF) should not be confused with acute liver failure (ALF), where a patient with ACLF presents with a distinct clinical feature than ALF and often requires LT as the only definitive treatment option. However, ACLF patients are generally not listed for the emergency LT due to advanced age, ongoing sepsis, multiple organ failures and active alcoholism. Then again, about 40% of the patients with ALF recover spontaneously with medical care and hence do not need LT. In between these all perplexities and contentions, it's critical to comprehend the clinical course of liver failure. In addition, physicians should also understand when it is necessary to enlist a patient for LT and which patient are likely to get benefit from LT. Thus, utilizing a "golden window" time for LT before the development of multi-organ failure. In this chapter, we focus on the current situation of LT for ALF and ACLF and further discuss the current decision making strategies used to indicate LT in this difficult clinical scenario.

Keywords: liver transplant, acute liver failure, acute-on-chronic liver failure, decompensated liver

1. Introduction

Decompensated liver or liver failure refers to the incompetence of the liver to accomplish its routine physiological functions. Generally, three forms of the liver failure have been outlined in the literature, i.e. acute liver failure (ALF), chronic liver failure (CLF) and more recently acute-on-chronic liver failure (ACLF) [1, 2].

ALF is described as an acute insult of the liver with encephalopathy and progressing worsening of the synthetic function of the liver (International normalized ratio (INR) ≥ 1.5) in a patient without cirrhosis or prior liver disease within 26 weeks of the onset of jaundice [3]. Whereas, CLF is broadly referred to the liver failure in end-stage liver diseases in the presence of cirrhosis. Cirrhosis is a dynamic chronic liver disease characterized by the histological progression of regenerative nodules encased by the fibrous tissues in response to chronic liver injury, that results to portal hypertension and liver failure [4]. Traditionally, the development of cirrhosis has been divided into two stages: 1. Compensated cirrhosis and 2. Decompensated cirrhosis [5]. Particularly, compensated cirrhosis endures between the onset of cirrhosis to the first considerable complication, that usually takes more than 10 years. However, most of the patients are usually asymptomatic or with minor complications. Further, the progression of compensated cirrhosis to decompensated cirrhosis occurs when there is development of ascites, variceal hemorrhage and/or hepatic encephalopathy and it is associated with a short-term survival. Nevertheless, the concept of the cirrhosis as an irreversible disease has been changed to the reversible disease, where the decompensated cirrhosis still can be reversed to the compensated cirrhosis or even to the pre-cirrhotic stage if the underlying disease is treatable [6]. Hence, it is apparent that the patients seldom dies as a result of an end-stage irreversible demolition of the liver. Relatively, in many patients, the reason for the death is an acute crumbling in their clinical condition advanced by a causative event, recently termed as ACLF [2]. ACLF is a syndrome characterized by an acute decompensation of the cirrhosis associated with the organ/system(s) failures and has a high 28 day mortality rate of 30–40% [7]. ACLF should not be confused with ALF, where a patient with ACLF present with a distinct clinical feature than ALF, and routinely require a different management approach. Liver transplant (LT) remains to be the only definitive treatment option for the patients with ACLF. However, the ACLF patients are generally not listed for an emergency LT due to an advanced age, ongoing sepsis, multiple organ failure, and active alcoholism. On the other hand, about 40% of the patients with ALF recover spontaneously with the medical care and hence do not need LT [8]. Therefore, it is extremely important to understand the clinical presentation and timing of the liver failure, so that the transplant surgeons can perceive when it is necessary to proceed with LT and which patients are likely to get benefit from LT.

In this chapter, we focus on the current scenario of LT for ALF and ACLF and further discuss the current decision making strategies used to indicate LT in this challenging clinical scenario.

2. Acute liver failure

ALF remains a rare condition that develops most commonly in the patients without pre-existing liver disease [9]. However, ALF is the matter of a concern for an apparent reason that it is typically associated with a high death rate. Often, the possible causes and precise mechanism of ALF are unspecified and uncertain [10]. Following the major hepatectomy, the patients with or without underlying liver disease, may typically develop a clinical syndrome similar to that of ALF. The clinical presentation is similar to that of the "small for size syndrome" following LT. These disorders are not considered inside the sphere of ALF, but rather are highlighted in some databases of ALF, for example, the European Liver Transplant Registry (ELTR). Moreover, the major liver injury has also been incorporated in ALF databases; however, it is not a cause of ALF except if there is loss of blood supply. Similarly, acute liver injury (ALI) should also be further differentiated from ALF, where the patients develop coagulopathy without vary in their level of consciousness.

Worldwide, viral hepatitis infection accounts for most cases of ALF. Where, hepatitis A and E are frequent causes in developing nations, while hepatitis B is a prevalent cause in some Asian and South American countries [11–13]. However, drug-induced ALF, particularly paracetamol induced ALF represents roughly half of the cases in the developed nations [14]. Moreover, ALF may likewise be diagnosed in the patients who earlier undiagnosed with Wilson's disease, vertically transmitted hepatitis B infection and autoimmune hepatitis, in whom concealed cirrhosis might be present, given the illness has been perceived for less than 26 weeks [15]. Then again, the patients with an acute alcoholic hepatitis, regardless of whether perceived for less than 26 weeks are considered to have ACLF since most have a protracted history of an excessive alcohol intake. ALF is commonly subdivided into hyperacute (<7 days), acute (>8 and <28 days), and subacute (>29 days and <26 weeks) contingent upon the time slipped by between the appearance of jaundice and progression of encephalopathy [16]. Nevertheless, the legitimate cut-off value of INR to define different subtype of ALF has not been documented yet.

The outcome of ALF is tough to predict. A few patients with ALF have fulminant progression, causing death without LT within a few days; others have fulminant progression of 2–4 weeks, and some patients even have an extended progression of 1–3 months. As stated earlier, the full recovery of damaged liver is conceivable. Thus, around 40% of the patients with ALF may recover completely without the need of LT [8]. Nonetheless, LT is shown to be a highly effective treatment for ALF where a mortality rate has been dropped down to 30% from 80% [17]. Despite that, a few issues still need to be taken into consideration while listing the patient with ALF for an emergency LT. 1. The hazard of LT for the patients who may recover spontaneously. 2. The hazard of not providing LT for the patients who really need it. 3. The survival benefit of the critically ill patients after LT.

2.1 Prognostic models and criteria for the selection of the patients with ALF for LT

Survival of the patients without LT varies upon the cause and subtypes of ALF [16]. In other words, the lessened the time spell between the commencement of jaundice and encephalopathy the better the prognosis. However, subacute liver failure where hepatic encephalopathy often develops just weeks after the beginning of jaundice has an especially low transplant-free survival and has a lower chance of spontaneous recovery in comparison to that of the hyperacute ALF [18]. In a study series of 300 consecutive ALF patients revealed that, ALF due to paracetamol and hepatitis A had an over 60% transplant-free survival rate, which was higher than that of ALF due to an idiosyncratic drug reaction, autoimmune hepatitis, hepatitis B virus, Wilson's disease, Budd-Chiari syndrome, and ALF due to an unknown cause [19]. Not too surprisingly, it has been found that the patients with lower grades of encephalopathy (**Table 1**) are more likely to have spontaneous recovery [20]. Additionally, it has also been revealed that the patients aged less than 10 or more than 40 years may have a lower probability of spontaneous recovery compared to those amidst these ages [19]. Furthermore, several other variables, for example gender, prothrombin time, renal function, Alpha-fetoprotein, arterial pH, factor V, serum lactate level, INR, liver biopsy, arterial ammonia level, and cell death marker level (CK 18/M65/M30) have been utilized to foresee the likelihood of recovery [21–24].

The choice to continue with LT relies on the likelihood of unconstrained hepatic recuperation. Nonetheless, the objective is to enhance the organ allocation system and accurate identification of the patients who are probably to get benefited from LT from those who are apparently going to recover spontaneously. Thus, avoiding the need of lifelong immunosuppressant in those patients who are supposedly to recover without LT. Additionally, reliable prognostic criteria are needed to make decisions on the proper timing of LT. Assuming that LT is performed too early, it might be performed when it is not needed, and if LT is delayed, there might be a higher risk of a poor outcome due to worsening condition of the patient.

Grade	Mental status	Asterixis	Neurological findings	EEG findings	Spontaneous recovery from ALF
Grade 0	Normal; potentially mild decrease in intellectual ability and coordination	Absent	Normal; if impaired psychomotor testing, consider minimal hepatic encephalopathy (MHE)	Normal	65–70%
Grade 1	Mild lack of awareness; hypersomnia, insomnia, or inversion of sleep pattern. Euphoria, depression, or irritability; mild confusion	May be present	Impaired addition or subtraction	Usually normal	
Grade 2	Lethargic; moderate confusion	Present	Disoriented; inappropriate behavior; slurred speech	Abnormal	
Grade 3	Somnolent but arousable; gross disorientation; bizarre behavior	Present	Muscular rigidity and clonus; hyperreflexia	Abnormal	40–50%
Grade 4	Coma	Absent		Abnormal	<20%

ALF, acute liver failure.

Table 1.
West-haven criteria for hepatic encephalopathy (HE).

Conditions such as hypoxic hepatitis, liver ischemia following liver trauma or liver surgery, haemophagocytic lymphohistiocytosis (HLH) precipitated by viral or fungal infections or hematological malignancy, and pregnancy related ALF are not an indication for emergency LT [18]. ALF may recover completely once the underlying causes are treated. However, in a condition like an autoimmune hepatitis patients should be listed for an emergency LT if the ALF fails to improve within 7 days [18]. Thus, the clinical skill of a doctor is important to make the proper decisions whether LT or other medical treatment is required in the above conditions.

Several prognostic models (**Table 2**) have been developed to predict the outcome and prognosis in the patients with ALF. The most broadly used criteria is the King's College Criteria for choosing the patients for LT [10, 15, 20, 25, 26]. Moreover, the Model for End-Stage Liver Disease (MELD) score, which is utilized to anticipate mortality in the patients with chronic liver disease, has additionally been tested to the patients with ALF [26]. Some other scores that may likewise anticipate mortality in the patients with ALF incorporates the Sequential Organ Failure Assessment (SOFA score) [27, 28], the Clichy criteria [26, 29, 30], Acute Physiology and Chronic Health Evaluation II (APACHE II) score [31], Acute Liver Failure Early Dynamic model (ALFED) [32], and the Acute Liver Failure Study

Criteria		Prognostic factors affecting outcome of patients	Sensitivity and Specificity
Clichy-Villejuif		• Coma and confusion (encephalopathy grade 3 or 4) and factor V < 20% of its normal value in patients under 30 years or • Coma and confuswion (encephalopathy grade 3 or 4) and factor V < 30% of its normal value in patients over 30 years	75% and 56% for Paracetamol induced ALF. 69% and 50% for non-Paracetamol induced ALF
King's College Hospital (KCH) criteria	Non-Paracetamol	• INR >6.7; or • Any three of the following: • Drug toxicity, regardless of whether it was the cause of ALF • Age < 10 or > 40 years • Jaundice to coma interval > 7 days • Bilirubin >300 µmol/L • INR >3.5	58% and 74%
	Paracetamol	• Arterial pH <7.3, or lactate >3 µmol/L after adequate volume resuscitation or • Encephalopathy grade 3 or 4 + creatinine >300 µmol/L + INR >6.5	90% and 69%
MELD score		• 10 × (0.957LnCreatinine[mg/L] + 0.378LnTotal Bilirubin[mg/dL] + 1.12LnINR + 0.643	79% and 71% for non-Paracetamol induced ALF
CK18/M65 MELD score		• 10 × (0.957LnCreatinine[mg/L] + 0.378LnM65[U/µl] + 1.12LnINR + 0.643	81.3% and 82.1%
ALF Early dynamic model (ALFED)		• ALFED score ≥ 4 on day 3	87.1% and 89.5%
Acute Liver Failure Study Group (ALFSG) index		• Admission coma grade • INR • Bilirubin • Phosphorus • log10 value of the apoptosis marker cleaved cytokeratin-18 (M30)	85.6% and 64.7%

MELD, Model for End-Stage Liver Disease.

Table 2.
Commonly used criteria as prognosis indicators in acute liver failure (ALF).

Group (ALFSG) index [33]. Sadly, none of these prognostic models have been found to be accurate. However, urgent LT is indicated in ALF where prognostic models suggest a high likelihood of death.

3. Acute-on-chronic liver failure

In the past ACLF has generally been used in critical care units to contemplate the patients who are on an artificial liver support a bridge to LT. As the name implies, the main concept in ACLF is an acute decompensation of the liver in a patient with chronic liver diseases and is associated with a high short-term mortality within 28 days [7]. Moreover, it is further characterized by hepatic and/or extrahepatic organ failure(s) [7, 34]. The pathophysiology of ACLF is yet largely not clear. Intense systemic inflammation and oxidative stress are considered to play a major role in the progression of the syndrome [35]. It has also been found that some patients with ACLF may recover with medical care to the state before onset of ACLF; and hence, such patients may not need emergency LT [36]. According to the CANONIC database, ACLF resolved or improved in 49.5% of the patients with medical treatment [37]. However, the prognosis is critical in the patients with no signs of improvement, and it is recommended that all the patients should be listed for LT before the development of multi-organ failure [36, 37]. Thus, these patients have a "golden window" period for LT before the development of extrahepatic organ failure(s) [38].

Numerous definitions of ACLF have been proposed [39, 40]; however, none of the definitions has acquired a global acceptance. The two most generally acknowledged ones are from an Asian Pacific Association for the Study of the Liver (APASL) [1] and the European Association for the Study of the Liver (EASL) Chronic Liver Failure (EASL-CLIF) consortium [2].

According to APASL consensus definition, ACLF can be defined as "an acute hepatic injury with an evidence of jaundice (a serum bilirubin of ≥5 mg/dl or ≥85 μmol/l) and coagulopathy (an INR of ≥1.5 or prothrombin activity of <40%) complicated within 4 weeks by clinical ascites and/or encephalopathy in a patient with previously diagnosed or undiagnosed chronic liver disease, i.e. with or without cirrhosis and is associated with a high short-term mortality within 28 days." [1] Criteria based on APASL definition, 90-day mortality is reported to be 13.1%. However, the APASL definition of ACLF had been developed on a speculative rather than the experimental basis.

The EASL-CLIF Acute-on-Chronic Liver Failure in Cirrhosis (CANONIC) study establish diagnosis of ACLF in the presence of organ failure as defined by the CLIF-Sequential Organ Failure Assessment (SOFA) score (**Table 3**) [41]. EASL-CLIF defines ACLF as "an acute deterioration of pre-existing chronic liver disease, usually related to a precipitating event [41] (**Table 4**) and associated with an increased mortality at 3 months due to multisystem organ failure" [2]. Currently, the time for the mortality has been defined by reducing to 4 weeks [42]. Overall, 28-day and 90-day mortality, according to EASL-CLIF criteria were reported to be 33% and 51%, respectively [2]. The EASL-CLIF definition is relevant to the patients with cirrhosis only (preferentially compensated or decompensated to represent chronic liver disease), in contrast, the APASL definition incorporates the patients with both cirrhotic and non-cirrhotic liver disease (yet not decompensated cirrhosis as interpreting "chronic"). Moreover, the EASL-CLIF definition also incorporates extrahepatic organ failures which are excluded by the APASL definition. Likewise, the precipitating events in the APASL definition are mainly hepatic in origin, though the EASL-AASLD definition incorporates sepsis [43]. The inconstancy in the standard definition and lack of an established management protocol for the ACLF patients further creates controversy among the physicians and surgeons.

As per EASL definition, the patients of ACLF are divided into four grades based on the numbers of organ failure (**Table 5**). Organ failures are a critical piece of prognosis

Organ/system	Subscore 1	Subscore 2	Subscore 3
Liver (bilirubin, mg/dl)	<6	≥6 to <12	**>12**
Kidney (creatinine, mg/dl)	<2	**>2 to < 3.5**	**≥3.5 or renal replacement therapy**
Brain (West-Haven grade for hepatic encephalopathy (HE))	Grade 0	Grade 1 or 2	**Grade 3 or 4**
Coagulation (INR)	<2.0	≥2.0 and < 2.5	**INR ≥ 2.5**
Circulation (mean arterial pressure)	≥70 mm/Hg	<70 mm/Hg	**Use of vasopressors**
Respiratory (PaO2/FiO2) Or SpO2/FiO2	>300 or > 357	≤300 and > 200 or > 214 and ≤ 357	**≤200 or ≤214**

Note: *Organ failures cutoff is highlighted in bold letters, Grade ACLF 1: patients with single kidney failure, patients with non-renal organ failure plus renal dysfunction (creatinine 1.5–1.9 mg/dl) and/or brain dysfunction (grade 1–2 HE). Grade ACLF 2: patients with 2 organ failures. Grade ACLF 3: patients with 3 or more organ failures.*

Table 3.
Organ failures and CLIF-C ACLF subscores.

Hepatic factors	Extrahepatic factors
• Flare-up or exacerbation of Hepatitis B virus infection	• Bacterial infection (Sepsis)
• Active alcoholism	• Gastrointestinal bleeding
• Superimposed Hepatitis A virus or Hepatitis E virus infections	• Surgery
• Drug-induced liver injury (DILI)	• Others non-identifiable factors
• Flare-up of autoimmune hepatitis or Wilson's disease	
• Transjugular intrahepatic portosystemic shunt (TIPS)	

Table 4.
Precipitating events for acute-on-chronic liver failure (ACLF).

in the patients with ACLF and with a higher number of organ failures (higher ACLF grades) the prognosis is poor [2]. It was found that the course of ACLF varies fast i.e. improves or deteriorates. Gustot et al. in his study demonstrated that the grade of ACLF can change unreasonably fast within 48 h in 40% of the patients, fast in between 3 and 7 days in approximately 14.7% of the patients and slowly in 8–28 days in 14.7% of the patients. Additionally, they also found that the ACLF grade at day 3–7 was better to anticipate the prognosis than the ACLF grade at the time of admission. Moreover, the ultimate ACLF grade remained the same in 81% of the patients after day 3–7 [37]. The characterization and subgroup division of ACLF on the basis of numbers of organ failure have led to an enhanced prognostic evaluation and provides a premise for determining selection criteria for LT and evaluation of those patients which may recover spontaneously with medical treatment only.

3.1 Prognostic models and criteria for the selection of the patients with ACLF for LT

It is critical to look at the course of ACLF, fail to improve organ(s) failure, despite maximal supportive treatment, especially by the day 3–7, is related to the

ACLF grade	Remarks
No ACLF	Patients who either: • Do not have any organ failure • Have a single organ failure that does not involve the kidneys with a serum creatinine level < 1.5 mg/dl and no hepatic encephalopathy • Have a single brain failure with a serum creatinine level < 1.5 mg/dl
ACLF grade 1	Patients with one of the following: • Single kidney failure • Single liver, coagulation, circulatory or respiratory failure that is associated with a serum creatinine level 1.5–1.9 mg/dl and/or grade 1 or grade 2 hepatic encephalopathy • Single brain failure with a serum creatinine level 1.5–1.9 mg/dl
ACLF grade 2	Two organ failures
ACLF grade 3	Three or more organ failures

Table 5.
Grades of acute-on-chronic liver failure (ACLF) based on the numbers of organ failure and types of organs.

bad prognosis, leading to the futility of care or consideration of an option for LT [39]. However, LT should not be done in a patient who may recover with medical treatment, and on the other hand, early LT should be considered in a patient with worsening or no improvement with the medical treatment before the development of multi-organ failure, thus considering the golden window period for LT [44].

Several prognostic models have been proposed in the last few years to better foresee the outcomes and prognosis of the patients with ACLF which includes, CLIF-C OF, CLIF-SOFA, SOFA, MELD, MELD-Na, and CTP scores [45].

As reported by CANONIC, the original grade of ACLF, the clinical course of ACLF, and a CLIF-C ACLF score (CLIF-C ACLF score combined CLIF-OF score with age and WBC count, calculator at www.efclif.com) appeared to precisely project the outcomes [2, 46]. CLIF-C ACLF score of up to 30 are steady with spontaneous recovery and the patients ought to have sequential evaluation regularly to decide if they are recovering. Moreover, with a score between 30 and 65, the patient is not likely to survive without LT; thus, such patients should be listed for an emergency LT without any delay taking other co-morbidities into the consideration for better outcomes. However, CLIF-C ACLF score over 65 brings up an issue of the futility to transplant and the secession of ongoing treatments [41]. In a study by Jalan et al. the CLIF-C ACLF score performed better when it was compared with the MELD, MELD-Na, and CTP scores [46].

In a recent study by Fangyuan et al. the group developed an HINAT ACLF model based on the APASL definition for ACLF due to hepatitis B reactivation, which includes five independent risk factors: Hepatic encephalopathy, international normalized ratio, neutrophil-lymphocyte ratio, age, and total bilirubin. According to this model, with the cutoff value of 4.6 for the HINAT ACLF score, the sensitivity and the specificity were 82.0% and 74.5%, respectively. Further suggesting that the performance of the HINAT ACLF score was significantly better than that of CLIF-C OF, CLIF-SOFA, SOFA, MELD, MELD-Na, and CTP scores [47].

Up to this point, MELD, MELD-Na and CTP scores, have been used to evaluate the prognosis of cirrhotic patients, with ACLF. However, these scores have limited value for foreseeing the prognosis in the ACLF patients, as these scores do not incorporate all the extrahepatic organ failures, which holds a critical effect on the prognosis of the ACLF patients.

In addition to the above prognostic models and scoring systems, various biomarkers have been identified that are found to reflect liver injury and multi-organ failure. These biomarkers might be of value in early diagnosis and progression prediction of ACLF if they can be incorporated with the CLIF-C ACLF score. Hyponatremia has appeared to have an independent prescient impact on 90 days survival [48] and copeptin concentrations in blood plasma showing changes in vasopressin level have appeared to ameliorate the ability of the CLIF-C ACLF score [49]. Additionally, urinary neutrophil gelatinase-associated lipocalin (N-GAL), plasma S100A8/A9 and soluble CD163 have also been shown to be increased in ACLF and correspond with the prognosis [50–52]. Apart from the above prediction models, the liver biopsy has also been found to be helpful in predicting the outcome and poor prognosis of ACLF, and further need for an early LT in these patients [53].

4. Liver transplantation in an acute decompensated liver failure

LT remains to be potentially the best treatment option, with better outcomes for patients with an acute decompensated liver failure. However, as stated earlier in this chapter, it is important to understand the clinical presentation of liver failure, where about 40% of the ALF patients show response to medical treatment and recover spontaneously and may not need LT. On the other hand LT remains to be the only definitive treatment option for the patients with ACLF.

4.1 Liver transplantation in ALF

LT has successfully reduced the mortality rate and improved overall survival in the patients with ALF, yet nearly 30% of the patients have to accept death without LT [54]. Outcomes of LT for ALF vary largely between different geographical regions and underlying etiologies behind ALF, where one-year survival ranges between 74% and 84% [54]. Regardless of this reality, results are better contrasted with a 64% oneyear survival depicted in the patients in ICU before LT, and to 54% seen in the patients on mechanical ventilation at the time of listing for LT [14, 55]. Most deaths for the patients with ALF are reported within the first 3 months of LT, generally because of neurological complications, multi-organ failure, and sepsis [56–58]. Additionally, efforts to identify the risk factors have been made, according to a study, recipient age above 50 years, history of life support, body mass index (BMI) above 30 kg/m^2, and serum creatinine of more than 2.0 mg/dL were the factors associated with a poor outcome [57]. Additionally, this study revealed that 5-year survival was significantly lower i.e. 42% for those patients meeting all these four factors compared to those with none i.e. 81% [57].

LT for ALF is most of the time and always done in an emergency situation. Usually, it is conceivable to transplant the ALF patient within 72 h after including the patient to the LT waiting list. However, due to the emergency situation, the likelihood of getting the best liver graft is minimized. In such situations, most of the time marginal grafts from the cadaveric donor are used as an option. It has been demonstrated that the utilization of these high-risk grafts may deleteriously affect post-transplant results and patient survival [59]. Apart from cadaveric LT living donor liver transplant (LDLT) is also commonly used, and the outcome of LDLT in the patients with ALF is found to be comparable to that of cadaveric LT [60]. Additionally, ABO-incompatible LT has also been tried out with a better survival outcome as compared with ABO-compatible LT. Indeed, ABO-incompatible LT has been found to be associated with a higher incidence of an antibody mediated rejection, Cytomegalovirus infection and biliary complications [61].

In ALF, the liver has the potential to regenerate by replication and differentiation of dormant hepatocytes and cholangiocytes [62] and thus the patients may recover without the need of a LT. Based on this, the concept of auxiliary partial orthotopic liver graft (APOLT) has been developed, where part of the native liver of the patient is left after performing a partial hepatectomy and a partial liver graft is transplanted in an orthotopic position [63]. In this way, the transplanted graft provides hepatic support to the patients while the native liver regenerates and recovers. Once the native liver returns to normal function, the dose of an immunosuppressant can be reduced slowly and finally withdrawn, further leading to the atrophy of the transplanted liver graft [64, 65]. However, the strategy of APOLT is challenging with the higher incidence of post-transplant complications [18, 66]. The native liver may not recover or regenerate significantly and may take a long time which depends upon multiple factors [66]. Therefore, use of APOLT should be limited to the patients with a high potential of liver regeneration, children, young adults, ALF due to hepatitis A virus and paracetamol poisoning [18, 66, 67]. Additionally, APOLT is not suitable for those patients with a high risk of brain death, high grade of hepatic encephalopathy, hemodynamically unstable patients who are on a higher dose of inotropes, or when ALF has advanced to a toxic liver syndrome [18, 66, 68].

4.2 Liver transplantation in ACLF

Taking LT for ACLF into consideration, most of the studies have indicated good results and equivalent survival rates in the patients transplanted for no ACLF [37, 69–73]; however, most of the earlier studies have not incorporated the patients with a high grade of ACLF i.e., with multi-organ failure. In the other studies, a poor outcome has been reported in the patients transplanted for the higher grades of ACLF [74–76], yet it still proves to be better than the survival rate of the patients without LT. In a similar context, a study by Gustot et al. demonstrated a survival rate of 80.9% at a half-year in the patients with ACLF grade 2 and 3, when contrasted with 10% in comparable grades of the ACLF patients who could not undergo LT [37]. Similarly, recent studies demonstrated a survival rate of >80% in the patients with ACLF grade 3 when contrasted with 7.9% in the controls, further suggesting a quick decision for LT to avoid high risk of mortality [74, 77].

It has been seen that the patients with ACLF showing development within 3–7 days are more likely to recover spontaneously [37, 38]. As reported by the CANONIC database, ACLF resolved or improved in 49.5% of patients with medical treatment. The resolution rates were 54.5%, 34.6% and 16% for ACLF grade 1, 2 and 3 respectively [37]. Additionally, the patients who fail to improve or with ongoing sepsis or multi-organ failure should immediately be considered for an early LT. However, precautions should be taken for the patients with respiratory failure and concomitant infection with multi-drug resistant organisms, due to risk of a higher rate of mortality and morbidity after LT [36, 77]. As of the dynamic nature of disease, the patients showing signs of the improvement in an early stage course of the disease may worsen later; thus, these patients should be monitored closely and listed for an early LT whenever required. Studies should focus on developing an ideal prognostic score, considering an extrahepatic organ failure, is needed to prioritize organ allocation on the waiting list, subsequently, to diminish delisting and mortality on the waiting list.

In the era of an organ shortage, living donor liver transplantation (LDLT) is the alluring choice with comparable results to the deceased donor liver transplantation (DDLT) in the high volume centers. Most of the LDLT related studies are carried out in Asian countries. However, it is not so famous in Western countries due to a higher rate of complications associated with it compared to DDLT [78–80]. Apart from this, the possibility of death of the donors and donor related complications clarified why LDLT has dropped in Western nations in the course of recent years [81, 82]. In a study from Hong Kong by Duan et al. reported, LDLT for the ACLF patients had a comparable result to DDLT in ACLF patients. Moreover, this study, concluded that the liver graft did not affect the outcome, where the overall 5-year survival rate was 74% for the LDLT for the ACLF patients [73].

Nonetheless, the objective of LT is not just to guarantee the patient's survival, yet additionally to offer an adequate quality of life. Sadly, the estimation of a quality of life in the general LT recipients, especially in the ACLF patients before LT, has not been thoroughly examined. For instance, stage 3 to 4 chronic kidney disease is developed in around 70% of the transplanted patients, with an increasing risk of end-staged renal disease needing a long-term hemodialysis or renal transplant within the initial 10 years after LT, that range somewhere between 3% and 9% [83, 84]. It has been found that, renal impairment is frequently encountered in the ACLF patients prior to LT, as is considered as an essential factor for the chronic kidney disease after LT [85]. Thus, the prevalence of end-staged renal disease after LT in the ACLF patients is as of now obscure and could enormously influence the post LT quality of life. Subsequently, a large database study is required on a long-term survival and quality of life after LT, not exclusively to affirm the prognosis of ACLF after LT, yet in addition to characterize rigorous selection benchmark that assist a good quality of life after LT.

5. Bridging to liver transplantation using an artificial liver support

In the past few decades, artificial liver support devices were developed to the point of being utilized as a supportive therapy option until LT (bridge to transplantation) and/or hepatic regeneration (bridge to recovery). The most commonly used devices are the Molecular Adsorbent Recirculating System (MARS), the Fractionated Plasma Separation, the Single-Pass Albumin Dialysis System (SPAD), and the Adsorption system [86]. However, it is still not clear that artificial liver support systems can help to bridge the patients with an acute decompensated liver to LT by eliminating toxins and enhancing liver functions [87, 88]. A meta-analysis of 12 randomized controlled trials utilizing different bioartificial liver support devices did not find a significant difference in the mortality rate when compared to the standard medical therapy [89, 90]. Nonetheless, a meta-regression, recommended that their impact rely on the type of liver failure. A 33% decrease in mortality was seen in the patients with ACLF, while no significant advantage was identified in those with ALF [90]. In contrary to this, a recent meta-analysis concluded that MARS and SPAD aid recovery of ALF [88].

6. When and whom to transplant?

It is important to identify those patients who may die without LT and those who may have a chance of spontaneous recovery. Thereby, dodging the need for lifelong immunosuppressant in the patients who are supposedly to recover without LT, and acting early for those who need LT. The early use of the selection criteria for LT in case of ALF or ACLF is mandatory in all the patients at the time of admission. Taking consideration of the dynamic nature of disease, all patients should be monitored closely and should be re-assessed time to time with the available prognostic criteria for any improvement or deterioration in the patient's status as discussed earlier in this chapter. Additionally, all patients presenting with an acute decompensated liver failure should be listed for an emergency or early LT to avoid any small margin of medical error, and thereby utilizing the "golden window" period for LT before the development of multi-organ failure (**Figure 1**).

LT is absolutely contraindicated in the patients with irreversible brain injury. Other conditions like vasoplegic shock with an increasing demand of vasopressor and uncontrolled ADRS are considered as a relative contraindication. Whereas, the bacteraemia is not considered as a contraindication providing that they can be treated with proper antibiotics. The concept of "Too Sick To Be Transplanted" is getting more popular in the recent years, considering the shortage of organs, the potential advantage of LT in the ALF or ACLF patients should likewise be adjusted against the requirement for proportioning of an insufficient resources [91, 92]. Similarly, the patients with alcohol-related liver disease (ARLD) should also be evaluated carefully for LT in light of constrained organ supply and the hazard that the ARLD liver recipient might return to risky drinking after LT [93]. Thus, the choice to proceed for

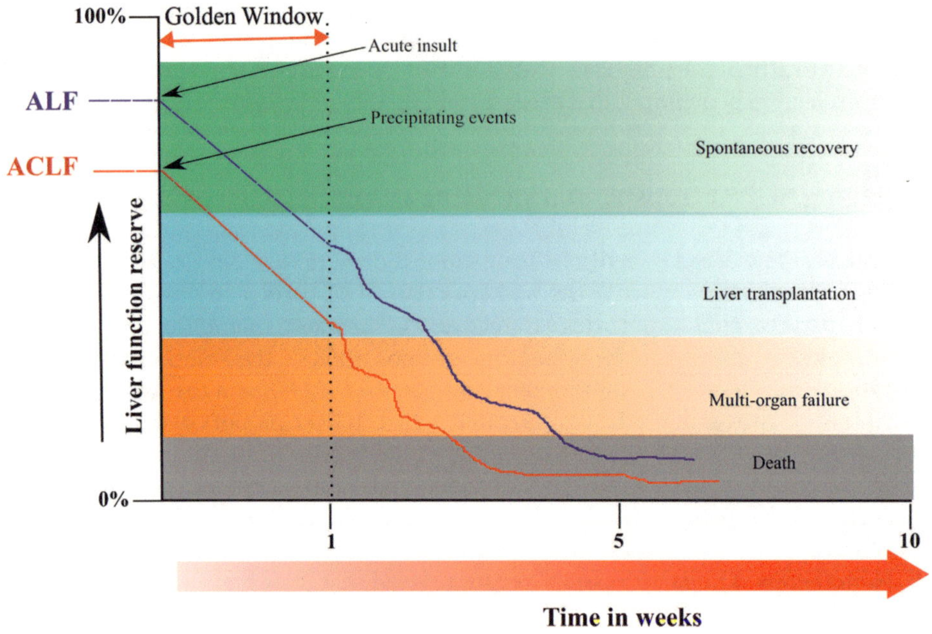

Figure 1.
The figure describes the an acute decompensated liver failure should be listed for an emergency or early LT in the first 1–2 weeks utilizing the "golden window" period for LT before the development of multi-organ failure.

LT should be discussed among all members of the multidisciplinary team taking both harm and benefit into the consideration.

Classically, disease severity scores like MELD have been used in several countries for an organ allocation. Nonetheless, the MELD score does not take an extrahepatic organ failure such as respiratory, brain, and circulatory failures into an account, thereby giving no preference for the patients with an acute decompensated liver failure. In a study, the patients undergoing LT with a MELD score > 30 had a 1-year overall survival rate of only 52.6% [94]. On the other hand, other studies have reported a poor outcome, particularly for those patients with a MELD score above 36 [95, 96]. Interestingly, Artru et al. showed a 1-year overall survival rate of 80% in the ACLF grade 3 patients with a median MELD score of 40 [74]. Thus, up to this point, there are no standard criteria and inadequate evidence to exclude too sick patients from a LT.

7. Conclusions

The choice to continue with LT for ALF relies on the likelihood of unconstrained hepatic recuperation and the underlying cause of ALF. Nonetheless, the objective is to enhance the organ allocation system and accurate identification of the patients who are probably to get benefited from LT from those who are apparently going to recover spontaneously. Thus, avoiding the need of lifelong immunosuppressant in those patients who are supposedly to recover without LT. Additionally, reliable prognostic criteria are needed to make decisions on the proper timing of LT. Assuming that LT is performed too early, it might be performed when it is not needed, and if LT is delayed, there might be a higher risk of poor outcome due to the worsening condition of the patient. In any case, the current evidence from the studies suggests that all the patients with ALF should be evaluated with an available criterion and should be listed for an emergency LT to avoid any small margin of medical error.

In spite of the assorted variety of early information on ACLF, two accord definitions by APASL and EASL have been developed recently, which exhibit two unique however coinciding circumstances. A few questions still have to be addressed in regards to which definition to utilize and whether there are contrasts inside a territory depending on the types of an underlying cause for ACLF found in each. Thus, albeit a few patients with an acute disintegration might not have ACLF initially at admission, considering ACLF as a dynamic syndrome that can improve or worsen during its course, clinicians should attempt to counteract patient vulnerability to new precipitating events and to identify the progression of ACLF immediately. ACLF patients are generally not listed for an emergency LT, regardless of the encouraging results. Thus, there is an urgent need for an ideal scoring system that can reveal the dynamic nature of ACLF and response to medical therapy.

Acknowledgements

This work was supported by grants from—National Key Research and Development Program (No. 2019YFC1316000), The National Natural Science Foundation of China (No. 81830089), Key Program of Medical Scientific Research Foundation of Zhejiang Province, China (No. WKJ-ZJ-1410), Zhejiang Provincial Program for the Cultivation of High-level Innovative Health talents.

Authors' contributions

(1) Conception and design: D. K. Yadav, and TB. Liang; (2) Writing of the manuscript: D. K. Yadav, R. K Yadav (3) Review of the manuscript: D. K. Yadav, R. K. Yadav, and TB. Liang.

Competing interests statement

The authors declare no competing interests.

Data availability

All the data supporting the results are shown in the paper and are available from the corresponding author upon request.

Author details

Dipesh Kumar Yadav[1,2,3,4,5], Rajesh Kumar Yadav[6] and Tingbo Liang[1,2,3,4,5]*

1 Department of Hepatobiliary Surgery and Liver Transplantation, The First Affiliated Hospital, Zhejiang University, Hangzhou, China

2 Zhejiang Provincial Key Laboratory of Pancreatic Disease, Hangzhou, China

3 Innovation Center for the Study of Pancreatic Diseases, Hangzhou, China

4 Zhejiang Clinical Research Center of Hepatobiliary and Pancreatic Disease, Hangzhou, China

5 Cancer Center, Zhejiang University, Hangzhou, Zhejiang, China

6 Department of Clinical Pharmacology, University of Louisiana at Monroe, USA

*Address all correspondence to: liangtingbo@zju.edu.cn

References

[1] Sarin SK, Kedarisetty CK, Abbas Z, Amarapurkar D, Bihari C, Chan AC, et al. Acute-on-chronic liver failure: Consensus recommendations of the Asian Pacific Association for the Study of the Liver (APASL) 2014. Hepatology International. 2014;**8**(4):453-471

[2] Moreau R, Jalan R, Gines P, Pavesi M, Angeli P, Cordoba J, et al. Acute-on-chronic liver failure is a distinct syndrome that develops in patients with acute decompensation of cirrhosis. Gastroenterology. 2013;**144**(7):1426-1437, 1437.e1421-1429

[3] Lee WM, Stravitz RT, Larson AM. Introduction to the revised American Association for the Study of Liver Diseases Position Paper on acute liver failure 2011. Hepatology (Baltimore, Md). 2012;**55**(3):965-967

[4] Schuppan D, Afdhal NH. Liver cirrhosis. Lancet. 2008;**371**(9615):838-851

[5] Gines P, Quintero E, Arroyo V, Teres J, Bruguera M, Rimola A, et al. Compensated cirrhosis: Natural history and prognostic factors. Hepatology (Baltimore, Md). 1987;**7**(1):122-128

[6] Ramachandran P, Iredale JP, Fallowfield JA. Resolution of liver fibrosis: Basic mechanisms and clinical relevance. Seminars in Liver Disease. 2015;**35**(2):119-131

[7] Arroyo V, Moreau R, Jalan R, Gines P. Acute-on-chronic liver failure: A new syndrome that will re-classify cirrhosis. Journal of Hepatology. 2015; **62**(Suppl. 1):S131-S143

[8] Reuben A, Tillman H, Fontana RJ, Davern T, McGuire B, Stravitz RT, et al. Outcomes in adults with acute liver failure between 1998 and 2013: An observational cohort study. Annals of Internal Medicine. 2016;**164**(11):724-732

[9] Bernal W, Wendon J. Acute liver failure. The New England Journal of Medicine. 2013;**369**(26):2525-2534

[10] Bernal W, Auzinger G, Dhawan A, Wendon J. Acute liver failure. Lancet. 2010;**376**(9736):190-201

[11] Jilani N, Das B, Husain S, Baweja U, Chattopadhya D, Gupta R, et al. Hepatitis E virus infection and fulminant hepatic failure during pregnancy. Journal of Gastroenterology and Hepatology. 2007;**22**(5):676-682

[12] Oketani M, Ido A, Tsubouchi H. Changing etiologies and outcomes of acute liver failure: A perspective from Japan. Journal of Gastroenterology and Hepatology. 2011;**26**(Suppl 1):65-71

[13] Mendizabal M, Marciano S, Videla M, Anders M, Zerega A, Balderramo D, et al. Changing etiologies and outcomes of acute liver failure: Perspectives from 6 transplant centers in Argentina. Liver Transplantation. 2014;**20**(4):483-489

[14] Lee W. Etiologies of acute liver failure. Seminars in Liver Disease. 2008;**28**(2):142-152

[15] Polson J, Lee W. AASLD position paper: The management of acute liver failure. Hepatology (Baltimore, Md). 2005;**41**(5):1179-1197

[16] O'Grady JG, Schalm SW, Williams R. Acute liver failure: Redefining the syndromes. Lancet. 1993;**342**(8866):273-275

[17] Akamatsu N, Sugawara Y, Kokudo N. Acute liver failure and liver transplantation. Intractable & Rare Diseases Research. 2013;**2**(3):77-87

[18] Wendon J, Cordoba J, Dhawan A, Larsen FS, Manns M, Samuel D, et al. EASL clinical practical guidelines on the management of acute (fulminant) liver failure. Journal of Hepatology. 2017;**66**(5):1047-1081

[19] Ostapowicz G, Fontana RJ, Schiodt FV, Larson A, Davern TJ, Han SH, et al. Results of a prospective study of acute liver failure at 17 tertiary care centers in the United States. Annals of Internal Medicine. 2002;**137**(12):947-954

[20] O'Grady JG, Alexander GJ, Hayllar KM, Williams R. Early indicators of prognosis in fulminant hepatic failure. Gastroenterology. 1989;**97**(2):439-445

[21] Samuel D, Ichai P. Prognosis indicator in acute liver failure: Is there a place for cell death markers? Journal of Hepatology. 2010;**53**(4):593-595

[22] Hoofnagle JH, Carithers RL Jr, Shapiro C, Ascher N. Fulminant hepatic failure: Summary of a workshop. Hepatology (Baltimore, Md). 1995;**21**(1):240-252

[23] Schmidt LE, Dalhoff K. Alpha-fetoprotein is a predictor of outcome in acetaminophen-induced liver injury. Hepatology (Baltimore, Md). 2005;**41**(1):26-31

[24] Clemmesen JO, Larsen FS, Kondrup J, Hansen BA, Ott P. Cerebral herniation in patients with acute liver failure is correlated with arterial ammonia concentration. Hepatology (Baltimore, Md). 1999;**29**(3):648-653

[25] Bernal W, Hyyrylainen A, Gera A, Audimoolam VK, McPhail MJ, Auzinger G, et al. Lessons from look-back in acute liver failure? A single Centre experience of 3300 patients. Journal of Hepatology. 2013;**59**(1):74-80

[26] Yantorno SE, Kremers WK, Ruf AE, Trentadue JJ, Podesta LG, Villamil FG. MELD is superior to King's college and Clichy's criteria to assess prognosis in fulminant hepatic failure. Liver Transplantation: Official Publication of the American Association for the Study of Liver Diseases and the International Liver Transplantation Society. 2007;**13**(6):822-828

[27] Craig DG, Zafar S, Reid TW, Martin KG, Davidson JS, Hayes PC, et al. The sequential organ failure assessment (SOFA) score is an effective triage marker following staggered paracetamol (acetaminophen) overdose. Alimentary Pharmacology & Therapeutics. 2012;**35**(12):1408-1415

[28] Craig DG, Reid TW, Wright EC, Martin KG, Davidson JS, Hayes PC, et al. The sequential organ failure assessment (SOFA) score is prognostically superior to the model for end-stage liver disease (MELD) and MELD variants following paracetamol (acetaminophen) overdose. Alimentary Pharmacology & Therapeutics. 2012;**35**(6):705-713

[29] Pauwels A, Mostefa-Kara N, Florent C, Levy VG. Emergency liver transplantation for acute liver failure. Evaluation of London and Clichy criteria. Journal of Hepatology. 1993;**17**(1):124-127

[30] Bernuau J, Goudeau A, Poynard T, Dubois F, Lesage G, Yvonnet B, et al. Multivariate analysis of prognostic factors in fulminant hepatitis B. Hepatology (Baltimore, Md). 1986;**6**(4):648-651

[31] Cholongitas EB, Betrossian A, Leandro G, Shaw S, Patch D, Burroughs AK. King's criteria,

APACHE II, and SOFA scores in acute liver failure. Hepatology (Baltimore, Md). 2006;**43**(4):881 author reply 882

[32] Kumar R, Shalimar SH, Goyal R, Kumar A, Khanal S, Prakash S, et al. Prospective derivation and validation of early dynamic model for predicting outcome in patients with acute liver failure. Gut. 2012;**61**(7):1068-1075

[33] Rutherford A, King LY, Hynan LS, Vedvyas C, Lin W, Lee WM, et al. Development of an accurate index for predicting outcomes of patients with acute liver failure. Gastroenterology. 2012;**143**(5):1237-1243

[34] Bajaj JS, O'Leary JG, Reddy KR, Wong F, Biggins SW, Patton H, et al. Survival in infection-related acute-on-chronic liver failure is defined by extrahepatic organ failures. Hepatology (Baltimore, Md). 2014;**60**(1):250-256

[35] Arroyo V, Moreau R, Jalan R. Acute-on-chronic liver failure. New England Journal of Medicine. 2020;**382**(22):2137-2145

[36] Choudhary NS, Saraf N, Saigal S, Soin AS. Liver transplantation for acute on chronic liver failure. Journal of Clinical and Experimental Hepatology. 2017;**7**(3):247-252

[37] Gustot T, Fernandez J, Garcia E, Morando F, Caraceni P, Alessandria C, et al. Clinical Course of acute-on-chronic liver failure syndrome and effects on prognosis. Hepatology. 2015;**62**(1):243-252

[38] Pamecha V, Kumar S, Bharathy KG. Liver transplantation in acute on chronic liver failure: Challenges and an algorithm for patient selection and management. Hepatology International. 2015;**9**(4):534-542

[39] Hernaez R, Sola E, Moreau R, Gines P. Acute-on-chronic liver failure: An update. Gut. 2017;**66**(3):541-553

[40] Arroyo V, Moreau R, Kamath PS, Jalan R, Gines P, Nevens F, et al. Acute-on-chronic liver failure in cirrhosis. Nature Reviews Disease Primers. 2016;**2**:16041

[41] Putignano A, Gustot T. New concepts in acute-on-chronic liver failure: Implications for liver transplantation. Liver Transplantation: Official Publication of the American Association for the Study of Liver Diseases and the International Liver Transplantation Society. 2017;**23**(2):234-243

[42] Jalan R, Stadlbauer V, Sen S, Cheshire L, Chang YM, Mookerjee RP. Role of predisposition, injury, response and organ failure in the prognosis of patients with acute-on-chronic liver failure: A prospective cohort study. Critical Care. 2012;**16**(6):R227

[43] Jalan R, Yurdaydin C, Bajaj JS, Acharya SK, Arroyo V, Lin HC, et al. Toward an improved definition of acute-on-chronic liver failure. Gastroenterology. 2014;**147**(1):4-10

[44] Sarin SK, Choudhury A. Management of acute-on-chronic liver failure: An algorithmic approach. Hepatology International. 2018;**12**(5):402-416

[45] Gustot T, Jalan R. Acute-on-chronic liver failure in patients with alcohol-related liver disease. Journal of Hepatology. 2019;**70**(2):319-327

[46] Jalan R, Saliba F, Pavesi M, Amoros A, Moreau R, Gines P, et al. Development and validation of a prognostic score to predict mortality in patients with acute-on-chronic liver failure. Journal of Hepatology. 2014;**61**(5):1038-1047

[47] Gao F, Sun L, Ye X, Liu Y, Liu H, Geng M, et al. Development and validation of a prognostic model for acute-on-chronic hepatitis B liver failure. European Journal of Gastroenterology & Hepatology. 2017;**29**(6):669-678

[48] Asrani SK, Simonetto DA, Kamath PS. Acute-on-chronic liver failure. Clinical Gastroenterology and Hepatology: The Official Clinical Practice Journal of the American Gastroenterological Association. 2015;**13**(12):2128-2139

[49] Kerbert AJC, Verspaget HW, Navarro ÀA, Jalan R, Solà E, Benten D, et al. Copeptin in acute decompensation of liver cirrhosis: Relationship with acute-on-chronic liver failure and short-term survival. Critical Care (London, England). 2017;**21**(1):321-321

[50] Ariza X, Graupera I, Coll M, Sola E, Barreto R, Garcia E, et al. Neutrophil gelatinase-associated lipocalin is a biomarker of acute-on-chronic liver failure and prognosis in cirrhosis. Journal of Hepatology. 2016;**65**(1):57-65

[51] Zhao R, Wu W, Zhou Z, Zheng X, Sun W, Shi Y, et al. Prognostic utility of novel biomarkers in acute-on-chronic liver failure (ACLF) associated with hepatitis B: A multicenter prospective study. Hepatology Research. 2019;**49**(1):42-50

[52] Singanayagam A, Nathwani R, Triantafyllou E, Patel VC, Dhar A, McPhail M, et al. PTH-106 plasma S100A8/A9: A novel mechanistic biomarker in innate immune activation in acute-on-chronic liver failure. Gut. 2018;**67**(Suppl. 1):A131

[53] Sarin SK, Choudhury A. Acute-on-chronic liver failure: Terminology, mechanisms and management. Nature Reviews. Gastroenterology & Hepatology. 2016;**13**(3):131-149

[54] Mendizabal M, Silva MO. Liver transplantation in acute liver failure: A challenging scenario. World Journal of Gastroenterology. 2016;**22**(4):1523-1531

[55] Freeman RB Jr, Steffick DE, Guidinger MK, Farmer DG, Berg CL, Merion RM. Liver and intestine transplantation in the United States, 1997-2006. American Journal of Transplantation: Official Journal of the American Society of Transplantation and the American Society of Transplant Surgeons. 2008;**8**(4 Pt. 2):958-976

[56] Tessier G, Villeneuve E, Villeneuve JP. Etiology and outcome of acute liver failure: Experience from a liver transplantation Centre in Montreal. Canadian Journal of Gastroenterology = Journal Canadien de Gastroenterologie. 2002;**16**(10):672-676

[57] Barshes NR, Lee TC, Balkrishnan R, Karpen SJ, Carter BA, Goss JA. Risk stratification of adult patients undergoing orthotopic liver transplantation for fulminant hepatic failure. Transplantation. 2006;**81**(2):195-201

[58] Germani G, Theocharidou E, Adam R, Karam V, Wendon J, O'Grady J, et al. Liver transplantation for acute liver failure in Europe: Outcomes over 20 years from the ELTR database. Journal of Hepatology. 2012;**57**(2):288-296

[59] Bernal W, Cross TJ, Auzinger G, Sizer E, Heneghan MA, Bowles M, et al. Outcome after wait-listing for emergency liver transplantation in acute liver failure: A single Centre experience. Journal of Hepatology. 2009;**50**(2):306-313

[60] Park SJ, Lim YS, Hwang S, Heo NY, Lee HC, Suh DJ, et al. Emergency adult-to-adult living-donor liver transplantation for acute liver failure in a hepatitis B virus endemic area. Hepatology (Baltimore, Md). 2010;**51**(3):903-911

[61] Yadav DK, Hua YF, Bai X, Lou J, Que R, Gao S, et al. ABO-incompatible adult living donor liver transplantation in the era of rituximab: A systematic review and meta-analysis. Gastroenterology Research and Practice. 2019;**2019**:8589402-8589402

[62] Fausto N. Liver regeneration and repair: Hepatocytes, progenitor cells, and stem cells. Hepatology (Baltimore, Md). 2004;**39**(6):1477-1487

[63] Rajput I, Prasad KR, Bellamy MC, Davies M, Attia MS, Lodge JP. Subtotal hepatectomy and whole graft auxiliary transplantation for acetaminophen-associated acute liver failure. HPB: The Official Journal of the International Hepato Pancreato Biliary Association. 2014;**16**(3):220-228

[64] Girlanda R, Vilca-Melendez H, Srinivasan P, Muiesan P, O'Grady JG, Rela M, et al. Immunosuppression withdrawal after auxiliary liver transplantation for acute liver failure. Transplantation Proceedings. 2005;**37**(4):1720-1721

[65] Quaglia A, Portmann BC, Knisely AS, Srinivasan P, Muiesan P, Wendon J, et al. Auxiliary transplantation for acute liver failure: Histopathological study of native liver regeneration. Liver Transplantation: Official Publication of the American Association for the Study of Liver Diseases and the International Liver Transplantation Society. 2008;**14**(10):1437-1448

[66] Rela M, Kaliamoorthy I, Reddy MS. Current status of auxiliary partial orthotopic liver transplantation for acute liver failure. Liver Transplantation: Official Publication of the American Association for the Study of Liver Diseases and the International Liver Transplantation Society. 2016;**22**(9):1265-1274

[67] Quadros J, Piedade C, Lopes MF. Auxiliary liver transplantation for management of acute liver failure in children—Systematic review. Transplantation Reviews (Orlando, Fla). 2021;**35**(4):100631

[68] Hessheimer AJ, Nacif L, Flores Villalba E, Fondevila C. Liver transplantation for acute liver failure. Cirugía Española (English Edition). 2017;**95**(4):181-189

[69] Chan AC, Fan ST, Lo CM, Liu CL, Chan SC, Ng KK, et al. Liver transplantation for acute-on-chronic liver failure. Hepatology International. 2009;**3**(4):571-581

[70] Liu C-L, Fan S-T, Lo C-M, Wei WI, Yong B-H, Lai C-L, et al. Live-donor liver transplantation for acute-on-chronic hepatitis B liver failure. Transplantation. 2003;**76**(8):1174-1179

[71] Wang ZX, Yan LN, Wang WT, Xu MQ, Yang JY. Impact of pretransplant MELD score on posttransplant outcome in orthotopic liver transplantation for patients with acute-on-chronic hepatitis B liver failure. Transplantation Proceedings. 2007;**39**(5):1501-1504

[72] Bahirwani R, Shaked O, Bewtra M, Forde K, Reddy KR. Acute-on-chronic liver failure before liver transplantation: Impact on posttransplant outcomes. Transplantation. 2011;**92**(8):952-957

[73] Duan BW, Lu SC, Wang ML, Liu JN, Chi P, Lai W, et al. Liver transplantation in acute-on-chronic liver failure patients with high model for end-stage liver disease (MELD) scores: A single center experience of 100 consecutive cases. The Journal of Surgical Research. 2013;**183**(2):936-943

[74] Artru F, Louvet A, Ruiz I, Levesque E, Labreuche J, Ursic-Bedoya J, et al. Liver

transplantation in the most severely ill cirrhotic patients: A multicenter study in acute-on-chronic liver failure grade 3. Journal of Hepatology. 2017;**67**(4):708-715

[75] Levesque E, Winter A, Noorah Z, Daures JP, Landais P, Feray C, et al. Impact of acute-on-chronic liver failure on 90-day mortality following a first liver transplantation. Liver International: Official Journal of the International Association for the Study of the Liver. 2017;**37**(5):684-693

[76] Agbim U, Sharma A, Maliakkal B, Karri S, Yazawa M, Goldkamp W, et al. Outcomes of liver transplant recipients with acute-on-chronic liver failure based on EASL-CLIF consortium definition: A single-center study. Transplantation Direct. 2020;**6**(4):e544

[77] Belli LS, Duvoux C, Artzner T, Bernal W, Conti S, Cortesi PA, et al. Liver transplantation for patients with acute-on-chronic liver failure (ACLF) in Europe: Results of the ELITA/EF-CLIF collaborative study (ECLIS). Journal of Hepatology. 2021;**75**(3):610-622

[78] Ghobrial RM, Freise CE, Trotter JF, Tong L, Ojo AO, Fair JH, et al. Donor morbidity after living donation for liver transplantation. Gastroenterology. 2008;**135**(2):468-476

[79] Marsh JW, Gray E, Ness R, Starzl TE. Complications of right lobe living donor liver transplantation. Journal of Hepatology. 2009;**51**(4):715-724

[80] Freise CE, Gillespie BW, Koffron AJ, Lok AS, Pruett TL, Emond JC, et al. Recipient morbidity after living and deceased donor liver transplantation: Findings from the A2ALL Retrospective Cohort Study. American Journal of Transplantation : Official Journal of the American Society of Transplantation and the American Society of Transplant Surgeons. 2008;**8**(12):2569-2579

[81] Hashikura Y, Ichida T, Umeshita K, Kawasaki S, Mizokami M, Mochida S, et al. Donor complications associated with living donor liver transplantation in Japan. Transplantation. 2009;**88**(1):110-114

[82] Kim PTW, Testa G. Living donor liver transplantation in the USA. Hepatobiliary Surgery and Nutrition. 2015;**5**(2):133-140

[83] Allen AM, Kim WR, Therneau TM, Larson JJ, Heimbach JK, Rule AD. Chronic kidney disease and associated mortality after liver transplantation--a time-dependent analysis using measured glomerular filtration rate. Journal of Hepatology. 2014;**61**(2):286-292

[84] Sola E, Gines P. Chronic kidney disease: A major concern in liver transplantation in the XXI century. Journal of Hepatology. 2014;**61**(2):196-197

[85] Khatua CR, Panigrahi S, Mishra D, Pradhan S, Sahu SK, Barik RK, et al. Acute kidney injury at admission is a better predictor of mortality than its persistence at 48 h in patients with acute-on-chronic liver failure. Journal of Clinical and Translational Hepatology. 2018;**6**(4):396-401

[86] García Martínez JJ, Bendjelid K. Artificial liver support systems: What is new over the last decade? Annals of Intensive Care. 2018;**8**(1):109

[87] He YT, Qi YN, Zhang BQ, Li JB, Bao J. Bioartificial liver support systems for acute liver failure: A systematic review and meta-analysis of the clinical and preclinical literature. World Journal of Gastroenterology. 2019;**25**(27):3634-3648

[88] Tandon R, Froghi S. Artificial liver support systems. Journal of

Gastroenterology and Hepatology. 2021;**36**(5):1164-1179

[89] Kjaergard LL, Liu J, Als-Nielsen B, Gluud C. Artificial and bioartificial support systems for acute and acute-on-chronic liver failure: A systematic review. JAMA. 2003;**289**(2):217-222

[90] Liu JP, Gluud LL, Als-Nielsen B, Gluud C. Artificial and bioartificial support systems for liver failure. The Cochrane Database of Systematic Reviews. 2004;(1):Cd003628

[91] Yadav DK, Zhang Q, Li BX, Liang T. Recent controversies in liver transplantation. Journal of Patan Academy of Health Sciences. 2020;**7**(2):98-102

[92] Weiss E, Saner F, Asrani SK, Biancofiore G, Blasi A, Lerut J, et al. When is a critically ill cirrhotic patient too sick to transplant? Development of consensus criteria by a multidisciplinary panel of 35 international experts. Transplantation. 2021;**105**(3):561-568

[93] Yadav DK, Zhang Q, Bai X, Li E, Liang T. Liver transplantation for alcohol-related liver disease (ARLD): An update on controversies and considerations. Canadian Journal of Gastroenterology and Hepatology. 2020;**2020**:8862152

[94] Weismüller TJ, Fikatas P, Schmidt J, Barreiros AP, Otto G, Beckebaum S, et al. Multicentric evaluation of model for end-stage liver disease-based allocation and survival after liver transplantation in Germany—Limitations of the 'sickest first'-concept. Transplant International. 2011;**24**(1):91-99

[95] Jacob M, Copley LP, Lewsey JD, Gimson A, Toogood GJ, Rela M, et al. Pretransplant MELD score and post liver transplantation survival in the UK and Ireland. Liver Transplantation: Official Publication of the American Association for the Study of Liver Diseases and the International Liver Transplantation Society. 2004;**10**(7):903-907

[96] Saab S, Wang V, Ibrahim AB, Durazo F, Han S, Farmer DG, et al. MELD score predicts 1-year patient survival post-orthotopic liver transplantation. Liver Transplantation: Official Publication of the American Association for the Study of Liver Diseases and the International Liver Transplantation Society. 2003;**9**(5): 473-476

Chapter 4

Liver Transplantation in Patients with Alcohol-Associated Liver Disease: Current Strategies and Future Perspectives

Federica Invernizzi and Marta Cilla

Abstract

Patients with alcohol-related liver disease (ALD) who receive a liver transplant (LT) reach a one-year post LT survival of 80–85%. The rule of abstinence from alcohol for 6 months before transplantation has been applied widely, but few data support the use of this rule as the only criterion for selecting LT candidates. Today, many liver transplant centers try to balance the duration of abstinence against the risk of death associated with the severity of ALD. Since 2011, an increasing number of papers suggests that transplantation without a specific period of abstinence (early LT) among patients with severe and nonmedical-therapy responder alcoholic hepatitis is an effective therapeutic strategy. Further data are needed to better define the selection of patients with ALD who have been abstinent for less than 6 months as suitable LT candidates and to improve the treatment of alcohol use disorder in those patients who have received a LT reducing the risk of alcohol abuse recurrence.

Keywords: alcohol-related liver disease (ALD), liver transplant (LT), early LT, alcohol abstinence, abuse recurrence

1. Introduction

Excessive alcohol use is the main cause of avoidable deaths in the USA with more than 95,000 deaths/y and 29 years lost per death [1].

Alcohol-associated liver disease (ALD) is the most frequent type of liver disease, existing on a spectrum that ranges from steatosis to steatohepatitis (with and/or without fibrosis), acute liver failure, severe alcoholic hepatitis (SAH) and cirrhosis [2].

Patients with severe ALD who do not respond to medical therapy have a poor prognosis and the only therapeutic option associated with a survival benefit is liver transplantation (LT).

To date, ALD is the most common defined cause for both LT (31%) and waiting-list diagnosis (31%) in the US [3]. As of 2019 in Europe, alcohol-related cirrhosis has become the most frequent LT indication, with graft survival rates of 78% at 3 years and 73% at 5 years post-transplantation [4].

The survival benefit of LT in patients with SAH and acute-on-chronic liver failure (ACLF) has been established [5–7]. Instead, survival benefit of transplantation versus no transplantation in patients with intermediate disease severity has not been proven [8, 9].

Nevertheless the consistent increase in the number of LT for AILD and its favorable outcome, less than 5–10% of potential candidates with this disease are listed for LT [10, 11].

Often alcoholics are held accountable for their disease. Moreover, these patients remain in situations of social and economic vulnerability that makes them susceptible to fall back into alcohol abuse. This has increased the disappointment towards their inclusion in transplant list.

Building on this, until some years ago, LT centers required a 6-month abstinence period to considerate patients for transplantation. However, data regarding the 6-month rule as a predictor of long-term sobriety are controversial [12].

Indeed, this period is arbitrary and has never been shown to affect survival after liver transplantation [13]. In additional, patients whose hepatitis is not responding to medical therapy have a 6-month survival rate of approximately 30%.

Since 2011, an increasing number of papers suggests that transplantation without a specific period of abstinence (early LT) among patients with severe and nonmedical-therapy responder alcoholic hepatitis is an effective therapeutic strategy [14].

Based on these data, transplant centres have gradually changed their procedures for handling of early liver transplantation. The percentage of early LT has tripled in France and has doubled in the USA over a period of almost 20 years [15]. However, before early LT can be expanded, it is vital to understand the long term survival and the factors associated with poor transplant outcomes.

2. Evaluation of alcohol-related liver disease patients for LT

In general, all LT candidates for ALD underwent careful evaluation by a multidisciplinary transplant committee, which consisted of transplant surgeons, herpetologists and licensed social worker. The latest guidelines in Europe and the USA have endorsed the integration of experts in addiction medicine in the process of assessing and managing alcohol use disorder in ALD during evaluation of individual patients for a transplant [16, 17].

Team members requested stringent selection for at least two reasons. First, donor grafts are not enough, second, in the allocation system based on MELD scores, patients with SAH and nonmedical-therapy response are like reaching the top of the transplant waiting list.

Foster *et al.* have proven that the length of pre-LT abstinence from ethanol alone is a poor predictor of post-LT abstinence when analyzed as a categorical variable like $<$ or $\geq$ 6-month abstinence and quantitative variable [18].

Furthermore, similar selection criteria are not applied to other LT candidates such as patients with nonalcoholic fatty liver disease (NAFLD) or intentional drug overdose, suffering from a similar addiction [19].

The transplant community must ensure that patient selection is fair and equitable and engenders continued faith and trust in the process. Appropriate safeguards are essential to excellent long-term outcomes comparable with other liver failure etiologies.

Wells *et al.* have proven that cirrhosis on explant pathology exceeded 95% in both early LT and standard LT groups, emphasizing that chronic liver disease is present in most patients despite an acute presentation. High rates of SAH on explant pathology was seen in 31% of patients in the standard LT group, despite patients reporting 6 months of abstinence [20].

This finding may reflect the heterogeneity in the duration of inflammation associated with alcohol or it may depend on ongoing alcohol abuse though patient-reported abstinence [20].

On the other hand, a meta-analysis of 92 studies involving ALD 8000 patients found that psychiatric comorbidities, abstinence for less than 6 months before transplantation, an unmarried status and smoking were predictive factors of alcohol relapse [21, 22].

Actually, transplantation community needs focus its interest from adherence to this arbitrary duration time of abstinence to identification of factors associated with poor post-transplant outcomes, post-transplant interventions that minimize relapse and strategies that treat relapse when it occurs. In additional, it's important to underline that the high prevalence of comorbidities in ALD candidates mandates a careful screening of extrahepatic comorbidities. Indeed, also other organs can be damaged by excessive drinking, for example alcohol-related acute pancreatitis is a relative contraindication to transplantation. A thorough cardiovascular and neurological assessment is required to exclude respectively cardiomyopathy and neuropathy alcohol-related.

All patients evaluated for liver transplantation should be screened also for malnourishment and sarcopenia. Sarcopenia is in fact a hallmark of frailty and functional decline and it has been recently identified as an independent predictor of waiting list mortality and worse post-transplant survival [23, 24].

Finally, alcohol-related cirrhosis is associated with an increased risk of hepatocellular carcinoma but also of other extrahepatic tumors, like cancer of the upper aerodigestive tract and, less often, colon and breast tumors [25].

3. Early vs. standard liver transplant

The treatment of patients with ALD has changed markedly over time. To ration organs, most programmes require a 6 month period of abstinence prior to evaluation of alcoholic patients, presumed to enable some patients to recover from their liver disease and identifying patients likely to maintain abstinence after LT [26].

However, data regarding the 6-month rule as a predictor of long-term sobriety are controversial [12]. Indeed, SAH is a life-threatening condition and corticosteroids for 1 month are the only approved medical treatment. Unfortunately, most alcoholic hepatitis deaths occur within 2 months and no pharmacological option has been proven efficient.

Starting from these data, 10 years ago Mathurin *et al.* selected 26 patients with severe alcoholic hepatitis at high risk of death (median Lille score, 0.88) and without severe coexisting or psychiatric disorders, with close family support and agreement for lifelong abstinence for early LT (median of 13 days after nonresponse to medical therapy). Mathurin *et al.* have shown that early transplantation was associated with higher cumulative 6-month survival rate compared with no early LT (77 ± 8% vs. 23 ± 8%, $P < 0.001$). Moreover, 2-years survival rates was higher in early-LT patients (hazard ratio, 6.08; $P = 0.004$). Finally, the assessment of alcohol relapse revealed that approximately 11% of patients remained daily alcohol drinker more than 3 years after LT [27]. Following this strategy, others Centers expanded access

Paper (authors and year)	Inclusion criteria	Exclusion criteria	Alcohol relapse rate (%)	1-year survival (%)
Mathurin P. [27] Dharancy S. (2020) [28]	• Medical therapy failure • First decompensating event due to severe AH • Close supportive family members and patient agreement to total abstinence • No psychiatric disorders	• Recent infection • Recent gastrointestinal bleeding	Clinical relevant: 10%	83%
Im G.Y. (2016) [29]	• Medical therapy failure • First decompensating event due to severe AH • Close supportive family members and patient agreement to total abstinence	• Concomitant chronic liver diseases • Concomitant hepatocellular carcinoma • Concomitant HIV • Severe comorbid conditions or psychiatric disorders	Any use: 22% Clinical relevant: 11%	89%
Weeks S.R. (2018) [30]	• Medical therapy failure • Close supportive family members and patient agreement to total abstinence • No coexisting psychiatric disorders • Patients with history of psychiatric symptoms included if psychiatric assessment demonstrated stably managed disease	• Concomitant liver disease • Concomitant hepatocellular carcinoma • Patients who received transplants previously	Any use: 28% Clinical relevant: 17%	97%
Lee B.P. (2018) [31]	• Age older than 18 years • First liver decompensating event due to severe AH • No prior diagnosis of chronic liver disease or episodes of AH • Strong social support by family and friends • Absence of severe comorbid medical disorders • Patient agreement to total abstinence	• Concomitant presence of other liver disease • HIV • Other contraindications to LT		
Germani G. (2021) [32]	• Age older than 18 years • Clinically diagnosed severe acute AH • Severe AH as the first liver decompensating event • Strong social support -Absence of severe comorbid medical disorders • Patient agreement to total abstinence	• Patient <18 years old • Concomitant presence of other liver disease • HIV	Any: 13%	100%

Paper (authors and year)	Inclusion criteria	Exclusion criteria	Alcohol relapse rate (%)	1-year survival (%)
Louvet A. (2022) [33]	• Aged 18 years or older. • High alcohol intake, clinical diagnosis of alcohol related hepatitis, hospitalized for less than 1 month • Maddrey score of 32 or higher at admission and poor response to medical management1 (Lille model score ≥ 0·45) or early • worsening of liver function despite an initial good therapeutic response (Lille model score < 0·45)	• HBsAg, hepatitis C virus, HIV antibodies, pregnancy, breastfeeding, evolving neoplasia likely to threaten 1-year outcome, and uncontrolled bacterial, fungal, parasitic, or viral infection	Any: 23%	89%

Table 1.
Selection criteria and outcomes in studies published on eLT for sAH.

to transplantation without 6-months rule among well-selected patients after careful assessment of their addiction profile **Table 1** [29, 31, 34].

Only 18 of 233 evaluated patients (7.7%) underwent transplant in the French cohort. In the initial US multicenter experience, the Accelerate trial, 36% of evaluated patients underwent transplant [31].

Recently, Herrick-Reynolds *et al* retrospectively analyzed data from largest single-center cohort of early LT for ALD to date to define patient, allograft, and relapse-free survival. Using standard LT as a comparison group, they also investigated the association of early LT with these survival outcomes [35].

In addition, a multicenter Italian study has shown that early LT significantly improves survival in SAH non-responding to medical therapy, when a strict selection process is applied. Overall, 6-, 12-, and 24-month survival rates were indeed 100% significantly higher in SAH candidated to early LT compared with non-responders to medical therapy who were denied LT (45%, 45%, and 36%, $p < 0.001$) [32].

Recently, Louvet *et al.* have conducted a multicentre, non-randomized, non-inferiority, controlled study in 19 French and Belgian hospitals. They cannot conclude non-inferiority in terms of rate of alcohol relapse post-transplant between early and standard LT proving that high alcohol intake is more frequent after early LT. On the other hand this prospective controlled study have confirmed the important survival benefit related to early LT for severe alcohol-related hepatitis [33].

Based on these data, despite the frequent use of the six-month rule, the United Network for Organ Sharing (UNOS), the International Liver Transplantation Society (ILTS) and the European Association for the Study of the Liver (EASL) Clinical Practice Guidelines on ALD and on LT did not endorse this measure as a formal recommendation [36].

4. Post-transplantation assessment

The proportion of patients returning to drinking any amount of alcohol range from 8 to 20% at 1 year post-transplantation and then gradually increase to 30–40% at 5 years post-transplantation [37].

DiMartini *et al.* have investigated patterns of alcohol use prospectively in long-term follow-up studies of LT patients and they observed no or minimal alcohol use over the follow-up period in 80% of patients [38].

Unfortunately, the reported rates of alcohol consumption after liver transplantation vary between studies because of the heterogeneous definitions used to classify recurrent drinking [26].

Available data indicate that, regardless of abstinence, a reduction in alcohol consumption is associated with a decrease in overall morbidity, mortality and health costs and an improvement in psychosocial status [39, 40].

Moreover, different studies have showed that only heavy or persistent drinking appear to be deleterious to the graft and long-term liver disease-related deaths in transplant recipients for ALD [41, 42].

Proceeding from this, the European Medicines Agency (EMA) and the US Food and Drug Administration (FDA) have defined drinking decreases a goal to assess efficacy in clinical trials. Accordingly, the EMA endorsed drinking risk levels reduction as outcome in alcohol pharmacotherapy trials in line with the WHO 4-category classification **Table 2** [39, 43].

Most trials focused in fact on abstinence goal until now, otherwise ongoing trials recognize alcohol level reductions as indicators of treatment outcome. This marks a revolution in the management of alcohol use defining drinking risk level reductions as a more worthwhile endpoint for ALD patients [44].

In a review of community-based epidemiology studies, alcohol dependence had the highest median untreated rate (78%) of the eight psychiatric disorders examined [45].

Reasons for these poor treatment rates may include the stigmatization of being labeled an alcoholic and individuals' resistance to stop drinking when treatment programs have traditionally focused on abstinence.

The link between alcohol abuse and poverty, discrimination, disadvantage and increased rates of psychological distress and are well known [46]. Alcohol related issues are best supported by a specialist team and the literature suggests specialized professionals embedded within the transplant team are the most effective in reducing post-transplant alcohol relapse and mortality [47, 48].

Psychosocial assessment is fundamental to establish predictive factors of unfavorable outcomes and associated possible intervention measures. Not adequate social assistance, ethanol/substance addiction and psychiatric problems may need heterogeneous strategies. Moreover, several patients can have multiple psychosocial problems that necessitate a coordinated pluridisciplinary approach [46].

Further research in this field is required to improve preoperative and postoperative patient-centred liver transplant outcomes.

Risk levels	Men	Women
Abstinence	0	0
Low risk	1–40	1–20
Medium risk	41–60	21–40
High risk	61–100	41–60
Very high risk	>101	>61

Table 2.
WHO risk levels of alcohol consumption, (g/day).

5. Conclusions and future directions

An increasing incidence of hospitalization for AH has been seen both in the United States and Europe, with a parallel increase in mortality rates in recent years.

Early LT for SAH is an emerging treatment option, although heterogeneities persist in national transplantation guidelines across countries.

We believe that a change in the approach to treating alcohol dependence is underway.

The core of the debate in the world of transplants is an ethical end cultural nature.

Is it right to donate a precious organ to patients who could resume post-LT alcohol addiction potentially resulting in the organ loss? The idea that patients without a proven period of alcohol withdrawal could damage to other patients on the waiting list has a potential detrimental effect on the willingness to donate organs.

Nevertheless, several studies have proven the important survival benefit related to early LT for SAH and these data have led to a gradual change in transplant centre practices.

Further progress is required to enhance the role of preoperative psychosocial counseling on the improvement of the recipient compliance and the addiction management after liver transplantation.

Moreover, the liver transplant candidate selection process needs to be standardized. The patient assessment need to focus on alcohol use disorder, coping skills and awareness and agreement to adhere to lifelong alcohol abstinence. Quality of affective relationship, presence or absence of caregiver support, good social and occupational functioning must be considered as critical factors.

Finally, we need prospective studies of interventions to treat alcohol dependence after transplantation focused on reduction in consumption of alcohol as opposed to abstinence.

Conflict of interest

The authors declare no conflict of interest.

Author details

Federica Invernizzi* and Marta Cilla
Center for Liver Disease, Division of Internal Medicine and Hepatology, IRCCS Ospedale San Raffaele, Milan, Italy

*Address all correspondence to: invernizzi.federica@gmail.com

References

[1] Mokdad AH, Ballestros K, Echko M, et al. The state of US health, 1990-2016: Burden of diseases, injuries, and risk factors among US states. JAMA. 2018;**319**:1444-1472

[2] Chacko KR, Reinus J. Spectrum of alcoholic liver disease. Clinics in Liver Disease. 2016;**20**(3):419-427. DOI: 10.1016/j.cld.2016.02.002

[3] 2019 Annual Data Report. Scientific Registry of Transplant Recipients. Available from: http://srtr.transplant.hrsa.gov/annual_reports/2019/Liver.aspx [Accessed June 20, 2021]

[4] Burra P, Senzolo M, Adam R, et al. Liver transplantation for alcoholic liver disease in Europe: A study from the ELTR (European liver transplant registry). American Journal of Transplantation. 2010;**10**:138-148

[5] Im GY, Cameron AM, Lucey MR. Livertransplantation for alcoholic hepatitis. Journal of Hepatology. 2019;**70**(2):328-334. DOI: 10.1016/j.jhep.2018.11.007

[6] Artru F, Louvet A, Ruiz I, et al. Liver transplantation in the most severely ill cirrhotic patients: A multicenter study in acute-on-chronic liver failure grade 3. Journal of Hepatology. 2017;**67**(4):708-715. DOI: 10.1016/j.jhep.2017.06.009

[7] Al-Saeedi M, Barout MH, Probst P, et al. Meta-analysis of patient survival and rate of alcohol relapse in liver-transplanted patients for acute alcoholic hepatitis. Langenbeck's Archives of Surgery. 2018;**403**(7):825-836. DOI: 10.1007/s00423-018-1720-z

[8] Poynard T, Naveau S, Doffoel M, et al. Evaluation of efficacy of liver transplantation in alcoholic cirrhosis using matched and simulated controls: 5-year survival. Multi-Centre group. Journal of Hepatology. 1999;**30**:1130-1137

[9] Poynard T, Barthelemy P, Fratte S, et al. Evaluation of efficacy of liver transplantation in alcoholic cirrhosis by a case-control study and simulated controls. Lancet. 1994;**344**:502-507

[10] Veldt BJ, Laine F, Guillygomarc'h A, et al. Indication of liver transplantation in severe alcoholic liver cirrhosis: Quantitative evaluation and optimal timing. Journal of Hepatology. 2002;**36**:93-98

[11] Watt KD, McCashland TM. Transplantation in the alcoholic patient. Seminars in Liver Disease. 2004;**24**:249-255

[12] Beresford TP, Everson GT. Liver transplantation for alcoholic liver disease: bias, beliefs, 6-month rule, and relapse — But where are the data? Liver Transplantation. 2000;**6**:777-778

[13] Tandon P, Goodman K, Ma M, et al. A shorter duration of pre-transplant abstinence predicts problem drinking after liver transplantation. The American Journal of Gastroenterology. 2009;**104**:1700-1706

[14] Antonini TM, Guillaud O, Dumortier J, Dharancy S, Saliba F, Mathurin P, et al; for Groupe de Recherche Français en Greffe de Foie (GReF2). Impact of a first study of early transplantation in acute alcoholic hepatitis: Results of a nationwide survey in french liver transplantation programs. Liver Transplantation. Jun 2018;**24**(6):841-844. DOI: 10.1002/lt.25039. Epub 2018 May 13. PMID: 29476690

[15] Bangaru S, Pedersen MR, MacConmara MP, Singal AG, Mufti AR.

Survey of liver transplantation practices for severe acute alcoholic hepatitis. Liver Transplantation. 2018;**24**:1357-1362

[16] Donnadieu-Rigole H, Jaubert L, Ursic-Bedoya J, et al. Integration of an addiction team in a liver transplantation Centre. Liver Transplantation. 2019;**25**:1611-1619

[17] Moriarty KJ. Collaborative liver and psychiatry care in the Royal Bolton Hospital for people with alcohol-related disease. Frontline Gastroenterology. 2011;**2**:77-81

[18] Foster PF, Fabrega F, Karademir S, Sankary HN, Mital D, Williams JW. Prediction of abstinence from ethanol in alcoholic recipients following liver transplantation. Hepatology. 1997;**25**:1469-1477

[19] Im GY, Cameron AM, Lucey MR. Liver transplantation for alcoholic hepatitis. Journal of Hepatology. 2019;**70**(2):328-334. DOI: 10.1016/j.jhep.2018.11.007

[20] Wells JT, Said A, Agni R, et al. The impact of acute alcoholic hepatitis in the explanted recipient liver on outcome after liver transplantation. Liver Transplantation. 2007;**13**(12):1728-1735. DOI: 10.1002/lt.21298), 10.1002/lt.21298)

[21] DiMartini A, Day N, Dew MA, et al. Alcohol consumption patterns and predictors of use following liver transplantation for alcoholic liver disease. Liver Transplantation. 2006;**12**:813-820

[22] Chuncharunee L, Yamashiki N, Thakkinstian A, Sobhonslidsuk A. Alcohol relapse and its predictors after liver transplantation for alcoholic liver disease: A systematic review and meta-analysis. BMC Gastroenterology. 2019;**19**:150

[23] Van Vugt JL, Levolger S, de Bruin RW, van Rosmalen J, Metselaar HJ, JN IJ. Systematic review and Meta-analysis of the impact of computed tomography-assessed skeletal muscle mass on outcome in patients awaiting or undergoing liver transplantation. American Journal of Transplantation. 2016;**16**:2277-2292

[24] Montano-Loza AJ, Duarte-Rojo A, Meza-Junco J, et al. Inclusion of sarcopenia within MELD (MELD-sarcopenia) and the prediction of mortality in patients with cirrhosis. Clinical and Translational Gastroenterology. 2015;**6**:e102

[25] Poschl G, Seitz HK. Alcohol and cancer. Alcohol and Alcoholism. 2004;**39**:155-165

[26] Mathurin P, Lucey MR. Liver transplantation in patients with alcohol-related liver disease: Current status and future directions. The Lancet Gastroenterology & Hepatology. 2020;**5**(5):507-514. DOI: 10.1016/S2468-1253(19)30451-0 PMID: 32277903

[27] Mathurin P, Moreno C, Samuel D, et al. Early liver transplantation for severe alcoholic hepatitis. The New England Journal of Medicine. 2011;**365**:1790-1800

[28] Erard-Poinsot D, Dharancy S, Hilleret MN, Faure S, Lamblin G, Chambon-Augoyard C, et al. Natural history of recurrent alcohol-related cirrhosis after liver transplantation: Fast and furious. Liver Transplantation. 2020;**26**(1):25-33. DOI: 10.1002/lt.25647. Epub 2019 Nov 22. PMID: 31562696

[29] Im GY, Kim-Schluger L, Shenoy A, et al. Early liver transplantation for severe alcoholic hepatitis in the United States a single-centreexperience. American Journal of Transplantation. 2016;**16**:841-849

[30] Weeks SR, Sun Z, McCaul ME, Zhu H, Anders RA, Philosophe B, et al. Liver transplantation for severe alcoholic hepatitis, updated lessons from the world's largest series. Journal of the American College of Surgeons. 2018;**226**(4):549-557. DOI: 10.1016/j.jamcollsurg.2017.12.044. Epub 2018 Feb 2. PMID: 29409981

[31] Lee BP, Mehta N, Platt L, et al. Outcomes of early liver transplantation for patients with severe alcoholic hepatitis. Gastroenterology. 2018;**155**:422-430

[32] Germani G, Angrisani D, Addolorato G, Merli M, Mazzarelli C, Tarli C, et al. Liver transplantation for severe alcoholic hepatitis: A multicenter Italian study. American Journal of Transplantation. Apr 2021;**22**(4):1191-1200. DOI: 10.1111/ajt.16936. Epub ahead of print PMID: 34954874

[33] Louvet A, Labreuche J, Moreno C, Vanlemmens C, Moirand R, Féray C, et al. Early liver transplantation for severe alcohol-related hepatitis not responding to medical treatment: A prospective controlled study. The Lancet Gastroenterology & Hepatology. May 2022;**7**(5):416-425. DOI: 10.1016/S2468-1253(21)00430-1

[34] Lee BP, Chen PH, Haugen C, et al. Three-year results of a pilot program in early liver transplantation for severe alcoholic hepatitis. Annals of Surgery. 2017;**265**:20-29

[35] Herrick-Reynolds KM, Punchhi G, Greenberg RS, Strauss AT, Boyarsky BJ, Weeks-Groh SR, et al. Evaluation of Early vs Standard Liver Transplant for Alcohol-Associated Liver Disease. JAMA Surgery. 1 Nov 2021;**156**(11):1026-1034. DOI: 10.1001/jamasurg.2021.3748. PMID: 34379106; PMCID: PMC8358815

[36] Karlsen TH, Sheron N, Zelber-Sagi S, Carrieri P, Dusheiko G, Bugianesi E, et al. The EASL-lancet liver commission: Protecting the next generation of Europeans against liver disease complications and premature mortality. Lancet. 2022;**399**(10319):61-116. DOI: 10.1016/S0140-6736(21)01701-3

[37] Tome S, Lucey MR. Timing of liver transplantation in alcoholic cirrhosis. Journal of Hepatology. 2003;**39**:302-307

[38] DiMartini A, Dew MA, Day N, et al. Trajectories of alcohol consumption following liver transplantation. American Journal of Transplantation. 2010;**10**:2305-2312

[39] Falk DE, O'Malley SS, Witkiewitz K, et al. Evaluation of drinking risk levels as outcomes in alcohol pharmacotherapy trials: A secondary analysis of 3 randomized clinical trials. JAMA Psychiatry. 2019;**76**:374-381

[40] Gastfriend DR, Garbutt JC, Pettinati HM, Forman RF. Reduction in heavy drinking as a treatment outcome in alcohol dependence. Journal of Substance Abuse Treatment. 2007;**33**:71-80

[41] Dumortier J, Dharancy S, Cannesson A, et al. Recurrent alcoholic cirrhosis in severe alcoholic relapse after liver transplantation: A frequent and serious complication. The American Journal of Gastroenterology. 2015;**110**:1160-1166

[42] Rice JP, Eickhoff J, Agni R, Ghufran A, Brahmbhatt R, Lucey MR. Abusive drinking after liver transplantation is associated with allograft loss and advanced allograft fibrosis. Liver Transplantation. 2013;**19**:1377-1386

[43] Hasin DS, Wall M, Witkiewitz K, et al. Change in non-abstinent WHO drinking risk levels and alcohol dependence: A 3 year follow-up study

in the US general population. Lancet Psychiatry. 2017;**4**:469-476

[44] Aubin HJ, Daeppen JB. Emerging pharmacotherapies for alcohol dependence: A systematic review focusing on reduction in consumption. Drug and Alcohol Dependence. 2013;**133**(1):15-29. DOI: 10.1016/j.drugalcdep.2013.04.025

[45] Kohn R, Saxena S, Levav I, Saraceno B. The treatment gap in mental healthcare. Bulletin of the World Health Organization. 2004;**82**:858-866

[46] Weiss E, Kabacam G, Gorvin L, Spiro M, Raptis DA, Keskin O, et al. The role of preoperative psychosocial counselling on the improvement of the recipient compliance and speed of recovery after liver transplantation - A systematic review of the literature and expert panel recommendations. Clinical Transplantation. Mar 2022;**6**:e14632. DOI: 10.1111/ctr.14632

[47] Addolorato G, Mirijello A, Leggio L, et al. Liver transplantation in alcoholic patients: Impact of an alcohol addiction unit within a liver transplant center. Alcoholism: Clinical & Experimental Research. 2013;**37**(9):1601-1608. DOI: 10.1111/acer.12117. Epub 2013 Apr 11. PMID: 23578009; PMCID: PMC4977094

[48] Donnadieu-Rigole H, Jaubert L, Ursic-Bedoya J, et al. Integration of an addiction team in a liver transplantation Center. Liver Transplantation; Nov 2019;**25**(11):1611-1619. DOI: 10.1002/lt.25641. Epub 2019 Oct 11. PMID: 31529607

Chapter 5

Analysis of the Behavior of Plasma Concentrations of Tacrolimus in Adult Patients with Liver Transplantation: Adverse Reactions and Drug Interactions and Their Relevance to Patient Safety

Victoria Fornari, Ana Fajreldines and Marcelo Pellizzari

Abstract

Organ transplantation is a medical treatment often used to restore the function of vital organs. Tacrolimus is one of the most widely used drugs in the immunosuppressive treatment of liver transplants. Aims: To analyze plasma concentrations of tacrolimus in adult liver transplant patients and to characterize adverse effects and drug interactions. Design: retrospective observational studies. The study included 32 patients, of whom 22 were male and 10 female. The average values and range of tacrolimus obtained showed a mean of 8.7 SD 3.2. Low values were found in seventy-five cases, with a percentage of 54.8%. The values within the expected had a frequency of fifty-three times with a percentage of 38.7%. Finally, the frequency of high values was nine times with a percentage of 6.5%. A total of 36 RAM types were found. It was determined that the majority of the ADRs were of moderate damage (13) of 46.4%, while 39.3% of the ADRs were of slight damage (11), 14.3% were of severe damage (4) and no ADR was incidental. Clinically relevant drug interactions in this group of patients were 16.7% contraindicated, 16.7% adjustments based on close follow-up, and 66.6% use with routine follow-up. Similar to the interactions present in the 2013 EMA data sheet. Plasma tacrolimus concentrations are within the range of 38.7% in male patients and 40.8% in female patients. 61.3% of male patients and 59.2% of female patients do not reach the expected tacrolimus plasma levels of 8.0–11.0 ng/ml, similar to those presented in the 2009 FDA data sheet. There were 220 ADRs in this sample of 32 liver transplant patients.

Keywords: tacrolimus, adverse drug events

1. Introduction

There are three forms of immunological rejection of liver transplantation, hyperacute, acute, and chronic rejection. Acute rejection of the transplanted liver is the most frequent form in which it is possible to act mainly with drugs [1]. Current immunosuppressive drugs are reducing their incidence from 60–80% in the 1960s–1980s to 30–50% today. From an immunological point of view, the liver is highly resistant to antibody-mediated attack and has a low rate of chronic rejection and high reversibility of acute rejection [2].

Immunosuppressant treatment is used in transplants to prevent acute or chronic graft rejection. The success of immunosuppression is finding the balance between preventing graft rejection and avoiding excessive suppression of individual's immune system.

Tacrolimus is one of the most widely used drugs in the immunosuppressive treatment of liver transplants, given that it has been shown to be more potent than cyclosporine, another drug used for the same purpose [3]. However, it has a wide intra-individual variability, which ranges between 10 and 40% according to the studies, and inter-individual, which has been estimated between 20 and 60% [4]. It has a bioavailability of 25–40% and, like cyclosporine, is metabolized by cytochrome P450 3A4. Its mechanism of action consists of binding to a cytoplasmic protein (FKBP) that inhibits calcineurin phosphatase [5], blocking the transcription factor for cytokine synthesis (IL-2, IL-4, IL-3, TNF, INF) and also the T-lymphocyte growth factor-beta. The most frequent adverse effects of tacrolimus are nephrotoxicity, neurotoxicity, hypertension, and diabetes, in addition to other, less relevant ones [6].

The advantage of tacrolimus is that it has great immunosuppressive power and, at low doses it is very effective, less toxic, and is generally used as monotherapy. One disadvantage is that it is a drug where the plasma concentration must be constantly monitored. Low levels of tacrolimus present the risk of graft rejection, while high levels produce greater toxic effects and increase the vulnerability of patients to infections and tumors. Another disadvantage of this drug is that it has numerous drug interactions because it is metabolized by the liver in cytochrome P450-3A4. Since many other drugs are metabolized by the same cytochrome, it gives rise to several interactions that may be clinically relevant and potentially serious [6].

2. Aims

To analyze plasma concentrations of tacrolimus in adult liver transplant patients and to characterize adverse effects and drug interactions.

3. Materials and methods

Design: a retrospective observational study on a random sample of adult patients with a history of liver transplantation.

Scope and period of the study: the study was conducted in a high-complexity hospital in Argentina in the period 2017–2018.

Study subjects: adult patients, who after their respective liver transplants, received treatment with tacrolimus as monotherapy or together with other appropriate drugs for their condition, if they needed it, according to the time elapsed from the transplant to the review of the data of this study. Only patients on immediate-release tacrolimus were assessed.

Sample: a sample of 32 patients was analyzed, and the sampling was done using the Excel formulas for W7 (probabilistic sample). The sample was randomly based on the total number of patients with liver transplantation and an indication for tacrolimus. The dose administered orally in adults was initially 0.10–0.15 mg/kg/day 24 hours after transplantation. After discharge, treatment with tacrolimus alone or in combination with other immunosuppressants was continued with doses varied according to clinical evaluation, rejection findings, and drug tolerance.

Data source: data were obtained from the electronic medical records (EHR) of each patient. Only relevant data regarding the patient's liver transplant, immunosuppressive treatment with tacrolimus alone or with other immunosuppressants, other concomitant medications, and present adverse effects were disclosed. The medical records began to be read from the date the patient was admitted to the hospital, even before the study period, since they are patients with longer treatment, and with multiple complications and hospitalizations.

4. Instruments

The monitoring of the plasmatic concentrations of tacrolimus obtained by means of dosages through the ELISA [7] technique in valleys after 10 days of therapy with tacrolimus was analyzed, and it was studied whether there was a readjustment of the dose if the patient was infra dosed or supra dosed to avoid graft rejection or increased frequency of adverse reactions. The expected range or optimal range of plasma dosages was considered to be between 8 and 11 ng/ml since this is the range estimated as optimal. In any case, any dosage above 11 or below was considered a deviation, since there are studies that indicate that concentrations between 5 and 8 ng/ml are associated with a lower severe toxicity profile and no graft rejection (Plinio, 2015).

Once the ADRs (adverse drug reactions) related to tacrolimus were classified, they were classified according to the Naranjo algorithm to find causality vs. chance. The algorithm questions were answered for each ADRs and a causality score was assigned to each one. Causality was classified as: definite (9 or more points), probable (5–8 points), possible (1–4 points), and doubtful (0 fewer points). See Annex I.

The 2003 WHO classification of drug safety was used to classify the harms of the ADRs found in this study according to whether they resulted in severe, moderate, slight, or incidental harm.

To determine the type of interactions, the Rothlin® database was used (See Annex II).

The preventability of the ADRs studies was analyzed using the Schumock [8] questionnaire.

5. Data collection

Data were collected in an excel spreadsheet, Windows 7. The software used for statistical analysis was SPSS ® 21 Software, ILLINOIS (USA). Laboratory variables, such as creatinine, TGP, TGO, age, sex, adverse effects, plasma concentrations of tacrolimus and interactions with concomitant medications, were studied.

Training of the data collector: the data were collected by the first author of this work, previously trained in intensive pharmacovigilance by the second author. Subsequently, a double check was made of a sample of 15 patients with tacrolimus, finding a weighted Cohen's Kappa of 0.73 (95% CI), a good agreement.

6. Results

The study included 32 patients, of whom 22 were male and 10 female. The percentage of men was 68.8% while that of women was 31.20%.

A total of 210 administered doses were studied, ranging from 0.5 mg every 12 hours to 8 mg every 12 hours.

320 trough concentrations in plasma were analyzed.

The average values and range of tacrolimus obtained showed a mean of 8.7 SD 3.2, and the distribution by sex was as follows (**Table 1**).

Low values were found in 75 cases, with a percentage of 54.8%. The expected values had a frequency of 53 times with a percentage of 38.7%. Finally, the frequency of high values was nine times with a percentage of 6.5%. A total of 36 RAM types were found.

In male patients, 23 different types of ADRs were recorded, 141 ADRs in total. The most frequent ADRs were gastrointestinal problems (34), hypertension (23), hyperglycemia (14), tremor (14), kidney failure (14), and muscle weakness (9). Those with the least frequency were oral ulcers (1), visual disturbances and discomfort (1), arthralgia (1), cytopenia (1), leukopenia (1), nocturia (1), and thrombocytopenia (1).

In female patients, 13 different types of ADRs were recorded, 78 ADRs in total. The most frequent were gastrointestinal problems (17), hypertension (13), renal insufficiency (8), and abnormal hepatogram (8). The least frequent were diarrhea (1), epigastric abdominal pain, and thrombocytopenia (1) (**Table 2**).

ADRs of probable causality were the ones with the highest percentage.

The most affected organ systems were blood and lymphatic system disorders (frequency 5–17.9%) and the least affected were cardiovascular disorders (frequency 1–3.6%), respiratory system disorders (frequency 1–3.6%), and disorders of the skin and appendages (frequency 1–3.6%). ADRs were also detected in the central and peripheral nervous systems (frequency 3–10.7%), gastrointestinal system (frequency 4–14.3%), general disorders of the whole organism (frequency 2–7.1%), metabolism and nutrition (frequency 3–10.7%), musculoskeletal system

Sex	Average	Range
Male	7.6 SD 2.1	2.2–18.8
Female	9.3 SD 5.4	2.6–26.1

Table 1.
Distribution by sex at range of tacrolimus.

Classification	Type of ADR	Percentage
Sure	6	14.3%
Probable	18	46.4%
Possible	10	28.6%
Improbable	3	10.7%
Total	28	100%

Table 2.
Frequency and percentage of adverse reactions to tacrolimus, according to causality using the Naranjo algorithm.

(frequency 3–10.7%), renal system (frequency 3–10.7%) and organs of vision (frequency 2–7.1%) (**Table 3**).

It was determined that the majority of the ADRs were of moderate damage (13) of 46.4%, while 39.3% of the ADRs were of slight damage (11), 14.3% were of serious damage (4), and no ADR was incidental.

Of the 30 patients who were administered by another type of medication in parallel to treatment with tacrolimus, it was determined whether there was a drug interaction between tacrolimus and the other drugs. It was found that 17 of the 30 patients, 56.7% received drugs that interacted pharmacokinetically with

ADR	Types of damage
Oral thrush	Mild
Visual disturbances, burning, and discomfort in the eyes	Mild
Anorexia	Mild
Arthralgia	Mild
Asthenia	Mild
Cramps	Mild
Headache	Mild
Cytopenia	Moderate
Muscular weakness	Moderate
Diarrhea	Mild
Dyslipidemia	Moderate
Epigastric abdominal pain	Mild
Edema in lower limbs	Moderate
COPD	Moderate
Fever	Mild
Altered hepatogram	Moderate
Hyperglycemia	Moderate
Hyperkalemia	Serious
Hypertension	Moderate
Urinary infection	Moderate
Renal insufficiency	Moderate
Leukopenia	Serious
Nocturia	Moderate
Plateletopenia	Serious
Gastrointestinal disorders	Moderate
Pruritus	Mild
Hypertensive retinopathy	Serious
Shaking	Moderate

Table 3.
Classification of ADRs according to the type of damage produced.

Patient	Interaction drug–drug
1	Tacrolimus vs. omeprazole
2	Tacrolimus vs. omeprazole
3	Tacrolimus vs. omeprazole and isoniazid
4	Tacrolimus vs. omeprazole
5	Tacrolimus vs. omeprazole
6	Tacrolimus vs. metoclopramide
7	Tacrolimus vs. omeprazole, everolimus, acetylsalicylic acid, and amlodipine
8	Tacrolimus vs. omeprazole
9	Tacrolimus vs. omeprazole and amlodipine
10	Tacrolimus vs. omeprazole
11	Tacrolimus vs. omeprazole y acetylsalicylic acid
12	Tacrolimus vs. omeprazole
13	Tacrolimus vs. omeprazole, everolimus and amlodipine
14	Tacrolimus vs. omeprazole and amlodipine
15	Tacrolimus vs. omeprazole
16	Tacrolimus vs. amlodipin
17	Tacrolimus vs. omeprazole

Table 4.
Drugs co-administered with tacrolimus.

Type of relevance according to drug interaction algorithm	Frequency	Percentage
Grade 1: do not use combination	1	16.7%
Grade 2: use, adjust guidelines, and follow the closest	1	16.7%
Grade 3: use with tracking	4	66.6%

Table 5.
Summary table of the frequency and degree of clinical relevance of tacrolimus drug interactions with other prescribed drugs.

Type of ADR	Frequency	Percentage
Preventables	7	25.0%
No preventables	21	75.0%

Table 6.
Summary table of the frequency and percentage of adverse reactions to tacrolimus according to their preventability.

Variable	OR_{aj}	IC95%	p Value
Sex	1.71	1.05–2.25	0.05
Impaired liver function	1.23	0.87–2.13	NS
Impaired kidney function	1.91	1.55–4.32	0.001
Presence of drug interaction	2.3	1.14–3.54	0.001
Age between 20 and 35 years	1.12	0.77–2.13	NS
Age between 36 and 55 years	1.25	0.87–1.69	NS
Between 56 and 65 years	1.09	0.98–2.31	NS
Age over 65 years	1.65	1.02–3.34	0.004
Presence of at least two dosages above the optimal values	3.24	2.45–3.78	0.002

Table 7.
Variables associated with the appearance of ADR.

tacrolimus, while, in the remaining 13 patients, 49.9% had no pharmacodynamic drug interactions (**Tables 4–6**).

In a logistic regression analysis, it was possible to analyze the association of various variables with the appearance of ADRs (**Table 7**).

7. Discussion

The mean plasma levels found coincided in a very similar way to the Varghese study with a very similar number of patients (8.5 vs. 8.3 in our study). The mean values to avoid manifestations of severe toxicity between 5–8 ng/ml were met in males, but not in females, where the standard deviation and the range were higher and wider, respectively.

Plasma tacrolimus levels in male patients averaged 7.6 ng/ml with a range of 2.2–18.8 ng/ml, while female patients averaged higher 9.3 ng/ml with a wider range of 2.6–26.1 ng/ml. In other words, the ranges of this study were wider than those recommended, and patients could be exposed to oscillations in plasma tacrolimus concentrations with their respective clinical consequences, but we see that in the ADR findings, the frequency of severe over the total found was 14.3%, with no relevant findings in terms of neurological consequences such as seizures, leukoencephalopathies, among others, as found in the study by Emiroglu et al. Which found a higher frequency of neurological ADRs, although pediatric patients participated in this study.

In this study, 54.8% of the men showed plasma concentrations lower than those recommended (8.0–11.0 ng/dL). Only 6.5% had concentrations higher than those recommended and 38.7% were found within the mentioned range.

40.8% of women showed optimal plasma concentrations (8.0–11.0 ng/dL). 19.7% had higher concentrations than recommended, and 39.5% had lower concentrations than recommended.

The range mentioned as optimal to avoid serious toxicity: 5–8 ng/ml, was present in 98 valleys measured in 14 patients; it is already seen that the inter- and intra-individual variability is high, as mentioned above. All RAM registered in this study are listed in the technical data sheet [9].

The causality of the ADRs recorded in this study was determined using the Naranjo algorithm. It was found that there were 14.3% of ADRs surely related to tacrolimus, 46.4% ADRs probably related, 28.6% possibly related, and 10.7% probably unrelated. These results were compared with the article, "Tacrolimus Toxicity with Minimal Clinical Manifestations: A Case Report and Literature Review" which discusses the toxicity of tacrolimus and compiles data from various sources of available literature about himself. Our study found similar results to those of this article [10].

There were 93.8%, 30 out of 32, patients with the administration of other medications along with tacrolimus treatment. The patients who presented drug interactions were 17 out of 30, 56.7%, who administered drugs together with tacrolimus. Drug interactions were found according to inter drug of rothlin drugs with omeprazole, isoniazid, metoclopramide, everolimus, acetylsalicylic acid, and amlodipine. Their degree of clinical relevance was then assessed using the clinically relevant drug interactions algorithm. One grade 1, 16.7% (everolimus), one grade 2, 16.7% (isoniazid), and four grade 3, 66.6% (omeprazole, metoclopramide, amlodipine, and acetylsalicylic acid) were found. In comparison, few drug interactions were found in the technical data sheet compared to the large number of interactions listed, there was only one contraindicated interaction, and the others were for use with caution and regular or careful monitoring. (Drug Inter, Rothlin Medicines, 2013).

Of the 28 ADRs, 7 of them, 25%, could have been prevented, while the remaining 21 ADRs could not.

The prevention of 25% of ADRs could have been achieved prior to subjecting the patient to treatment with tacrolimus. One way to prevent these ADRs would have been to treat the patient with medication prior to or together with the administration of tacrolimus, carrying out early monitoring of tacrolimus concentrations in plasma, and above all, educating the patient in a more systematic way and with a method that the patient can understand without giving rise to doubts, or erroneous interpretations that could lead to problems related to the medication.

The variables sex, impaired renal function, elderly patients, patients with some levels out of range, and the presence of drug interaction are the variables found to be related to the appearance of adverse events in this sample of patients.

The 2013 EMA data sheet states that drug interactions and patients older than 65 years increase the probability that tacrolimus values are outside the range of 8.0–11.0 ng/dL.

Similar results were found in the article "Adverse Drug Events in Hospitalized Patients with Chronic Kidney Disease" by Yahaya Hassan, which mentions that renal impairment increases the incidence of ADRs compared to patients without RF .

The study by Bates DW, Miller EB, Cullen DJ, et al., "Patient Risk Factors for Adverse Drug Events in Hospitalized Patients", as in this study, establishes that patients who present drug interactions are more likely to manifest reactions adverse than patients without drug interactions [5].

The study "Adverse drug reactions in older people" by Tangiisuran C coincides with the results found in this study that elderly patients are more likely to manifest ADRs than younger patients.

We have found, in this study, a wide range of plasmatic concentrations of tacrolimus in 32 patients; this variability has been evaluated by multiple published studies, and added to this, its narrow therapeutic index and the potentiality of its multiple pharmacological interactions, the control of concentrations blood pressure of tacrolimus is useful in optimizing therapy and dosing regimen design.

8. Conclusions

Plasma tacrolimus concentrations are within range by 38.7% in male patients and 40.8% in female patients. 61.3% of male patients and 59.2% of female patients do not reach the expected tacrolimus plasma levels of 8.0–11.0 ng/ml. Similar to those presented in the 2009 FDA data sheet.

There were 220 ADRs in this sample of 32 liver transplant patients, and the most common ADRs were gastrointestinal problems, hypertension, renal failure, tremor, and hyperglycemia.

There are several variables associated with the appearance of adverse effects.

Patients treated with tacrolimus as immunosuppressive therapy for liver transplantation should be closely monitored. Plasma concentrations of the same should be maintained within the normal or optimal range, 8.0–11.0 ng/ml in plasma to avoid rejection of the transplanted liver, infections due to excess immunosuppression, and preventable adverse reactions.

Author details

Victoria Fornari[1*], Ana Fajreldines[2] and Marcelo Pellizzari[1]

1 Hospital Universitario Austral, Argentina

2 Hospital Alemán, Argentina

*Address all correspondence to: vfornari@gmail.com

References

[1] Amariles, Pedro, Giraldo, Newar Andrés, Faus, Maria José. Drug interactions: Approach to establish and evaluate their clinical relevance. Clinical Medicine (Barcelona). 2007:129(1). Available from: http://www.elsevier.es/es-revista-medicina-clinica-2-articulo-interacciones-medicamentosas-aproximacion-establecer- evaluate-13106681. [Accessed August 27, 2015]

[2] Catalan Association of Malalts d'Hepatitis. Liver Transplant. 2015. Available from: http://asscat-hepatitis.org/situacion-mundial-de-las-hepatitis/. [Accessed May 24, 2015]

[3] Astella Pharma Inc. A Study to Assess the Pharmacokinetics of a Modified-Release Tacrolimus Based Immunosuppression Regimen in Stable Liver Transplant Patients. 2013. Available from: https://clinicaltrials.gov/ct2/show/study/NCT00282243?term=tacrolimus+liver+transplantation&rank=28&sect=X43r0156. [Accessed: August 31, 2015]

[4] Backman L, Nicar M, Levy M, et al. FK506 through Levels in Whole Blood and Plasma in Liver Transplant Recipients: Correlation with Clinical Events and Side Effects. Department of Surgery, Baylor University Medical Center. 1994. Available from: http://www.ncbi.nlm.nih.gov/pubmed/7509516. [Accessed: April 20, 2015]

[5] Bates DW, Miller EB, Cullen DJ, et al. Patient risk factors for adverse drug events in hospitalized patients. Archives of Internal Medicine. 1999;**159**(169):2553-2560. www.ncbi.nlm.nih.gov/pmc/articles/PMC2855002. [Accessed: September 18, 2015]

[6] Bilbao I, Margarit C. Immunosuppression in Liver Transplantation (chapter 48). 2005. Available from: http://www.cirugiasanchinarro.com/sites/default/files/gonzales48.pdf.[Accessed: August 30, 2015]

[7] Bioacademy. Immunoenzymatic assays <ELISA>. 2015. Available from: http://www.bioacademia.com.mx/miembros/tecnologia/0003.html.Casola. [Accessed: May 31, 2015]

[8] Schumock GT, Thornton JP. Focusing on the preventability of adverse drug reactions. Hospital Pharmacy. 1992;27:538. Available from: http://www.researchgate.net/publication/13178574. [Accessed: September 4, 2015]

[9] European Medicines Agency (EMA). Avdagraf: EPAR Product Information, Annex I: Technical Sheet or Summary of Product Characteristics 2013. Available from: http://www.ema.europa.eu/docs/es_ES/document_library/EPAR_-_Product_Information/human/000712/WC500022234.pdf. [Accessed: on April 28, 2015]

[10] Haroon, Nivin, Sinhg, Atul, Bhar, Zeenat Yousuf. Tacrolimus toxicity with minimal clinical manifestations: A case report and literature review. American Journal of Therapeutics. 2015;1-4:3. Available from: http://www.ncbi.nlm.nih.gov/pubmed/25730156. [Accessed: 1 de septiembre, 2015]